> "Beautiful, yet surprisingly simple. My first time making broth, but certainly not the last."

> "Tangy, spicy and very easy to follow. Superb."

> "Satisfying mouthfuls of autumnal flavours."

> "Good enough to serve in a restaurant."

Fatima Sonia
Bandeiro
Faye Morris
Fiona Bates
Fiona Campbeell Hall
Fiona Christoffers
Fiona Haywood
Fiona Hutchinson
Fiona Kelsey Quayle
Fiona Lander
Fiona Merwood
Fiona Scott

Ginny Christy
Glenda Alquicer Barrera
Guy Tucker
Gwyneth Ashcroft

Hannah Burton
Hannah Greenwood
Hatti Crawford
Hazel Cumberland
Heather Jill Hickson
Heather Leeson
Heather Mozley
Heather Smith

Gabby Rouse
Gabriella Aquilina
Gareth Brock
Geeta Patel
Gemma Costello
Geraldine Nolan
Geraldine Short
Gill Bailey
Gill Evans
Gill Hartley
Gill Methven
Gillian Page
Gina Fletcher
Gini Woodward

Helen Beckett
Helen Ford
Helen French
Helen Hunter
Helen Kennedy
Helen Knowles
Helen Murray
Helen Woolley
Helena Bevis
Hélène Flint

Ian Rogerson
Ildiko Edge
Inez McGinley

Jackie Caffrey
Jackie Elms
Jacky Houghton
Jacqueline Darby
Jacqueline Durbin
Jacqui Cox
Jacqui Dean
Jacqui Hardy
Jade Bootsma
Jaimee Behan
Jan Curle
Jan Hoare
Jan Thomas
Jane Clayton
Jane Edwards
Jane Lillington
Jane Mork
Jane Page
Jane Paul
Janet Ayscough
Janet Churchward
Janet Pauline Nicholls
Janice Tidmarsh
Janie Alexander
Jasmine Greene
Jazmin Andrews
Jean Bacon

Jemma MacDonald
Jennifer Nicholson
Jenny Lawrence
Jenny Long
Jenny Simpson
Jenny Stone
Jessica Dahlgren
Jessica Higham
Jessica Saunders
Jill Lambeth
Jill Riddiford
Jo Campbell
Jo McCollin
Jo Osborne

Joanne Fleming
Joanne Garcia
Joanne Gauci
Joanne Rushworth
Johanna Havercroft
John & Pat Beeson
Josephine Isaac
Josie Gadsby
Josie McKinnon
Juanita Tulett
Judith Morrison
Judith Stone
Judy Murray
Jules Fell
Julia Reilly
Julia Wilks
Julie Banks
Julie Byers
Julie Denison
Julie Malmborg
Julie Palfrey
Julie Tipper
Juliet Alison Locke
Julieta Medina
  Franqueira
Juliette Culver
Juliette Ward

Karen Burroughs
Karen Falcone
Karen MacGregor
Karen Preece
Karen Reed
Karen Salamon
Karen Wyett
Karin Ayres
Karin Orchard
Karina Montagni
Kate Ale
Kate Carr

DR RUPY AUJLA

COOKS

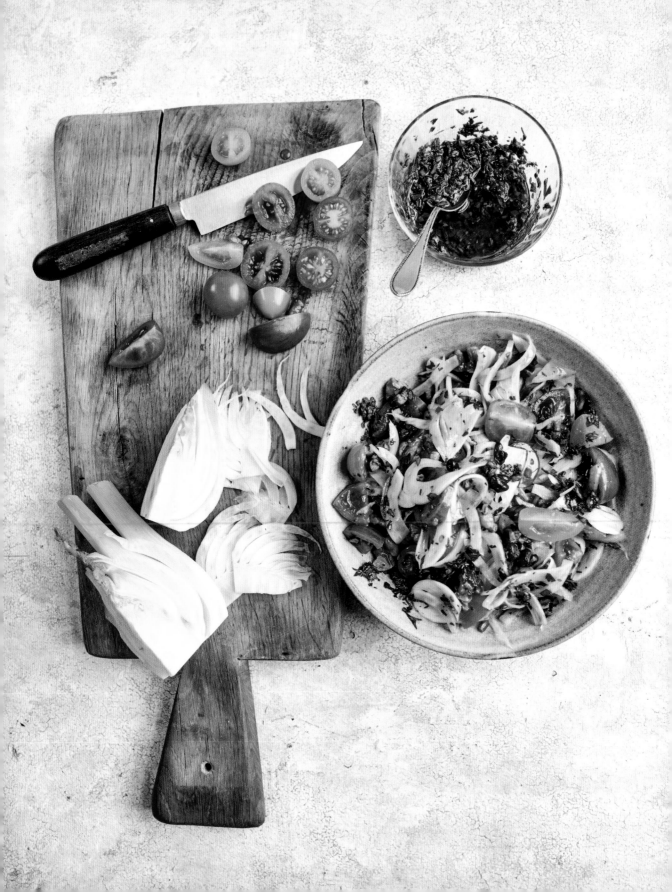

DR RUPY AUJLA

COOKS

Healthy * Easy * Flavour

Photography by David Loftus

EBURY
PRESS

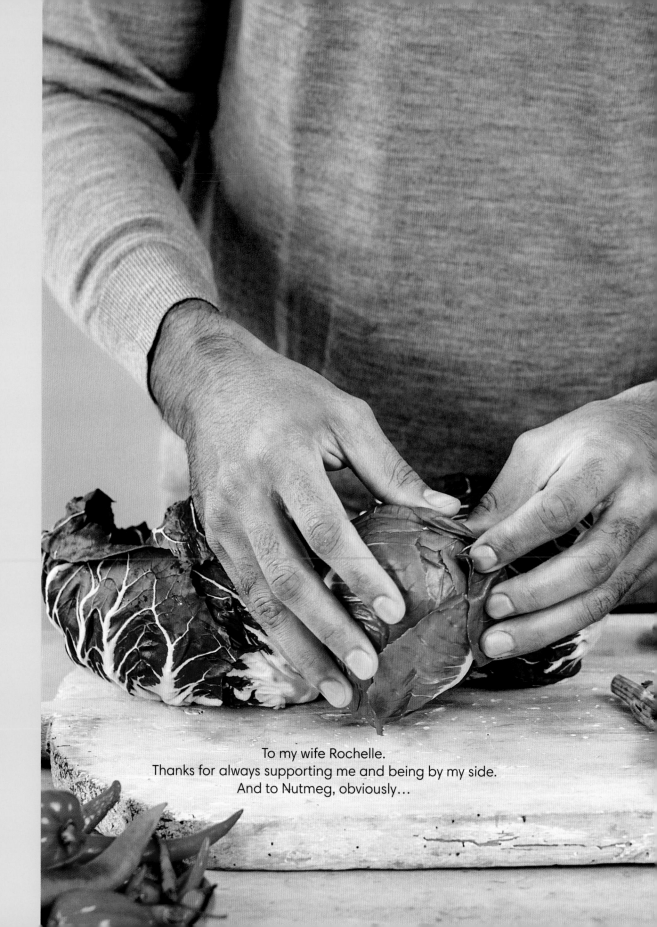

To my wife Rochelle.
Thanks for always supporting me and being by my side.
And to Nutmeg, obviously…

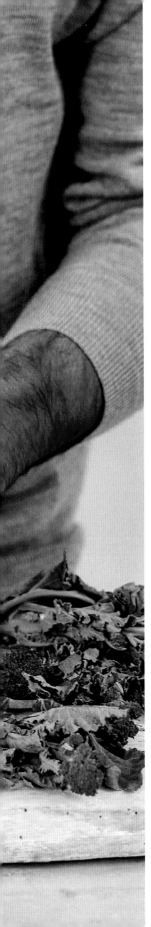

CONTENTS

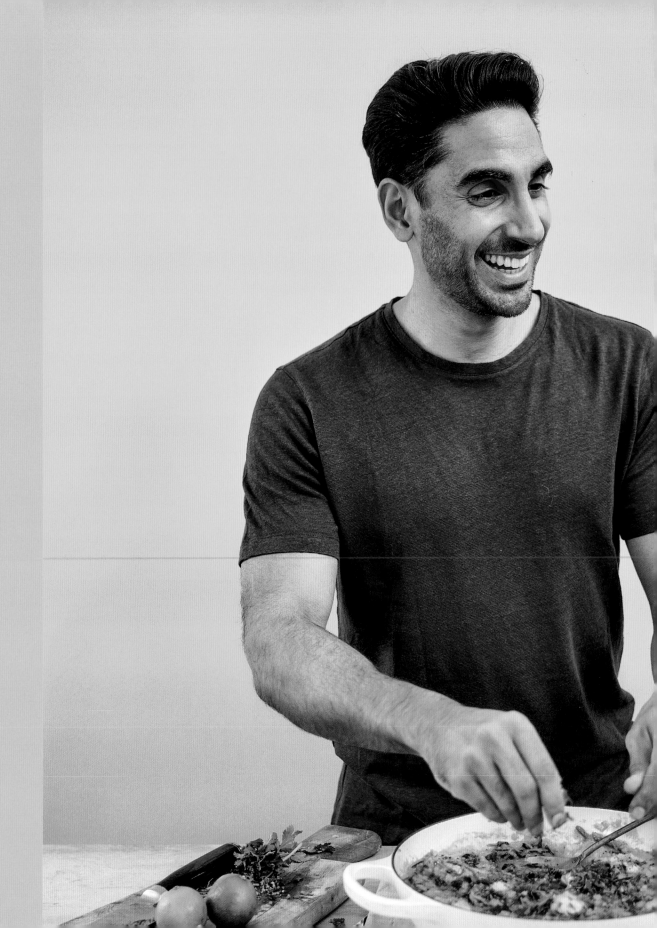

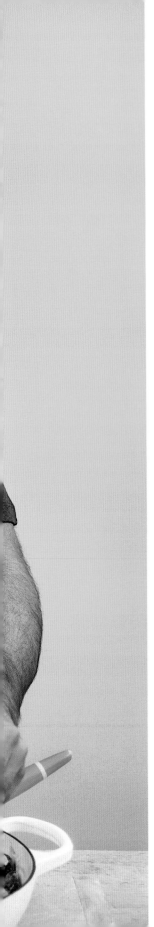

INTRODUCTION

I'm Dr Rupy, an NHS GP, food writer and advocate of nutritional medicine. My mission is to help everybody leverage the incredible power of food and lifestyle medicine to support their wellbeing, daily performance and prevent ill health. After reading hundreds of academic papers, studying for a masters in nutrition and seeing thousands of patients in clinic for over a decade, it's clear to me that the best thing we can all do for our health is to improve our diet and maintain a healthy way of eating every day. And that's the crux of it. Eating well, every day.

We've been led to believe that the secret to good health lies in a set of specific ingredients and restrictive diet plans, when in reality the health benefits of food rely on eating consistently well daily. Good food doesn't have to be expensive or out of the ordinary; on the contrary, healthy eating should be enjoyable and achievable over the long term. And that's where the informative content on my podcast and delicious recipes within this book can help.

People are driven to eat well for different reasons. Perhaps your family doctor has told you to cut out certain foods for health reasons. Maybe you feel sluggish and overtired most days and somebody suggested it could be your diet. You may have recently started a family and have resolved to finally look after yourself so you can keep up with the kids, or perhaps you feel slower, less responsive, less vivacious with each birthday and this realisation has spurred you on to take control of your wellbeing. Regardless of your motivation for picking up this book, my promise to you is this: I will help you eat better every day.

Over the past decade, I've explored nutritional science from many angles, speaking to communities within medicine, nutrition and wellness, as well as thousands of people who want to become more knowledgeable about nutritional medicine. Nothing excites me more than knowing my recipes are having a positive impact on people's health across the globe. And this is just the start.

MY INFLUENCES

In addition to the science of nutritional medicine that underpins every one of my recipes, my Indian culinary heritage has been the gateway to my food-as-medicine ethos. At the heart of Punjabi cuisine is an emphasis on vegetables and beans, cooked with freshly ground spices to create subtly perfumed dishes. Alongside the basic principle of less meat and more vegetables, the foundations of an ancient Ayurvedic diet – which I grew up with – still form the basis of my cooking.

Beyond the clichés of turmeric milk and garam masala are the lesser-known Ayurvedic practices that most Indians have come across. The importance of a balanced, flavourful plate that includes salty, sweet, sour, pungent, astringent and bitter – the nutritional elements needed for complete nourishment and absorption. The focus on gut health to maintain equilibrium across all bodily systems. The use of rejuvenating plants (rasayanas) in both culinary and medicinal contexts to support everything from pain management, brain function and enhanced virility. While I question the evidence for and efficacy of many Ayurvedic practices, the principles of mindset, movement, rest and nourishment as a formula for health are hard to argue against. I've been on the receiving end of many an 'I told you so' from family members whenever research emerges on the importance of traditional herbs, like ashwagandha, or fermented foods.

From my Indian heritage, personal health journey, academic studies and clinical practice, these influences have culminated in a unique perspective on food, lifestyle and medicine. My experience as a GP in the NHS has helped me distil this complex information into relatable daily practices shared in clinic, where I draw from both ancient and modern approaches to medicine. In trying to inspire my multi-cultural patient population to eat better, I'm tasked with making dietary suggestions that are not only actionable but also relatable to them.

It's a job I've come to adore as it allows me to explore a wealth of cuisines from across the globe. When you dig a little deeper and examine the traditional diets of Mexico, Korea, the

Levantine region and Italy, to name a few, it all feels strangely familiar to my experiences from childhood. Corn and beans spiced with jalapeños, sour kimchi paired with earthy sesame paste and short-grain rice, and the combination of aubergines, garlic and hazelnuts enlivened by the tang of ruby red sumac. Those salty, sweet, sour, pungent, astringent and bitter elements that I used to associate solely with an Ayurvedic method of cooking appear to be present across the traditional diets of many other cultures.

Regardless of heritage, our ancestors cracked the code to good health and wellbeing through food. This may sound odd coming from a conventionally trained doctor who is used to working in Accident and Emergency, but we need to take notice of these ancient practices and realise that the foundation for our health starts on our plate. We need not restrict ourselves to an Ayurvedic, Japanese Washoku or even Mediterranean-inspired cuisine. Inherent in traditional diets from across the world are common threads of dietary principles that, when examined through the lens of recent discoveries, all appear to support health.

What is even more fascinating is that the science is now proving how traditional diets are so healthful and why we should be adopting more of these approaches to promote wellbeing and curb chronic disease. As such, my recipes skip through cuisines from across continents and showcase ingredients from many countries that all happen to combine to create exceptionally healthy and delicious dishes. Hopefully these recipes will entice you to take full advantage of the natural medicines that line the grocery aisles.

FLAVOUR & FUNCTION

As a doctor obsessed with the functional benefits of food, you might think that I would ignore the beauty of ingredients and focus solely on their medicinal properties. But food is so much more than just a collection of calories and micronutrients consumed to support the functioning of our bodies. Recipes are reflections of people's cultures, histories and memories. The pleasure derived from sitting around a table and experiencing someone's hospitality, or even enjoying the self-care of a midweek meal prepared for one, is something I don't ever want to lose in a book because it's focused on healthy eating.

Dr Rupy Cooks honours the joy derived from cooking and the rich traditions of dishes, while blending that with the science of food as medicine. I assure you that every meal you prepare from this book is truly good for your health and respects the heritage of its inspiration: each dish is a marriage of flavour and function.

Ingredients can take your palate on a vibrant adventure. With colour, texture and flavour, my recipes teach you how healthy eating can be accessible and delicious. In addition, I aim to convince you that a diet designed to support your wellbeing doesn't need to conform to a Eurocentric menu, which is common in 'healthy' cookbooks. Regardless of what cuisine you prefer, each dish is fulfilling and good for you. Dishes from India, Ghana and Latin America can all be just as delicious and health-promoting as Mediterranean food. The health stamp is not reserved for specific cuisines, and I'm passionate about showcasing the potential benefits of recipes across all cultures.

My job is to highlight the functional benefits of ingredients used within recipes to inspire and guide you towards a healthier, more delicious way of eating every day. I also don't want this to come across too puritanical either. At work, everybody reels in horror when they see me eating a handful of indulgent chocolates from the nurses' station. The fact of the matter is this: food is not just one of the most significant health and wellbeing interventions, it's also one of the most important sources of pleasure. It's glorious, comforting, enticing and rewarding. Eating and sharing food is one of the most enjoyable aspects of life – something I don't want anyone to forget.

WHY YOU SHOULD JOIN ME

My ultimate goal is to welcome you on a journey of eating well for life, without you ever necessarily realising that you're eating healthily. This will be food you want to share with family and friends, food your children will enjoy and approve of, food that's easy and simple to make without exorbitant expense or time needed to seek out the ingredients.

It's also important that we're honest with ourselves about the potential value of food. Rather than using brassica vegetables as a garnish to complement a healthy-looking meal, I use ingredients in the necessary quantities to ensure they actually deliver on their proposed benefits. For that reason, each meal contains three or more portions of fruit, vegetables, nuts or seeds per person, which is in line with new research that recommends the 'doses' of foods we need to sustain and optimise our health.

By respecting the basics of cooking and principles for building flavour, this book for everyday wellness is going to be pivotal for your health in a way that won't feel punitive or restrictive. With each delicious recipe you make, you'll be effortlessly supporting your heart, brain, immune system, skin and more. This book is for people who love food and want to live better. I promise you, the two are not mutually exclusive and I hope at the end of each recipe you make from this book, you'll be reminded of that.

For now, let's start off with the basic principles of what makes food so nourishing. I'll teach you the fundamentals of healthy eating distilled from research studies that have influenced my recipes and this book will guide you through the basics of increasing vegetables, limiting refined carbohydrates and sugar, increasing fibre and focusing on plant-based proteins. You'll begin to realise how each meal is carefully crafted to deliver on the food-as-medicine philosophy as well as making it super-simple to achieve and maintain this habit one delicious plate at a time.

IT STARTS
IN THE GUT

Even in solitude, you're in the company of trillions of friends who have been with you since birth. Your inner community of microbes are the reason you're alive today, reading the pages of this book. They've grown up with you, co-evolved with your immune system, nourished you and protected you.

This complex community of microbes is your gut microbiota, including largely bacterial species, but also viruses and fungi, that form their respective microbiome, virome and mycobiome systems. These micro-organisms exist inside us all, mostly populating our large intestine, but also the surface of our skin, eyes and lungs. These microbes are tasked with releasing micronutrients from food, creating fatty acids that nourish gut cells, maintaining an inflammation balance to support immune function, producing the neurochemicals that keep us calm and happy... The list goes on.

If you've recently read any scientific paper or popular nutrition news, you will have noticed that the power of food and its ability to protect our health seems to be centred around how we can impact and modulate the gut, this 'forgotten organ'. It's very much an interdependent, reciprocal relationship we have with our microbes and one that we must nurture for a well-functioning body and mind as it impacts our mental health, cardiovascular health and more. Essentially, a happy gut means a happy brain, strong immune system, efficient metabolism and glowing skin.

This is where food comes in. Many factors impact the health of our microbiota – genetics, stress, exercise, antibiotics, environmental pollution – but diet is arguably the most adjustable and effective intervention within our daily control, which can rapidly change this ecosystem for better or for worse. In this section, I focus on what the science determines as a pattern of eating that aligns with a healthy gut microbe population, as well as some categories of ingredients that will help your microbes thrive. Instead of considering this as yet another tedious list of foods you 'have to have' in your diet, think about these ingredients through the lens of beautiful dishes and cuisines that traditionally contain them.

I could write an entire book on gut health, explaining the intricacies of each microbial species, how they impact each of our organs, how we measure microbial health through testing and what the future holds. Instead, I want to keep it super simple and focus on the three key principles that deliver most bang for your buck. There are a wide range of ingredients that support gut health, but stick with these at each mealtime and I guarantee you'll be effortlessly supporting your magnificent microbes, which is aligned with optimal physical and mental health.

Prebiotics

Often sidelined in favour of sexier-sounding probiotics are the humble prebiotics. To explain what they are, let's consider everyone's favourite celebratory drink, Champagne. The saying goes, all Champagne is sparkling wine, but not all sparkling wine is Champagne. Using this analogy, all prebiotics are fibre, but not all fibres are prebiotics.

Prebiotics are specialised types of fibre that we ourselves cannot digest but have unique properties in building up our microbes, conferring tangible health benefits to us. When consumed even in small amounts (as little as 5g per day), these fibres stimulate the growth of specialised intestinal bacteria, like *bifidobacteria* and *lactobacilli*, which have been recognised to enhance mood, improve immune health and even strengthen bones.

When I consider ingredients that contain prebiotic fibres, like leeks, garlic, asparagus, artichokes, chicory root, bananas, barley and rye, I think of exquisite traditional dishes: Greek horta, Carciofi alla Romana, French-style endive and walnut salad, asparagus risotto, chapatis made with a variety of milled grains. The use of health-promoting ingredients is encoded in the DNA of many traditional recipes, which is easy to recognise once you know what you're looking for. Woven throughout this book, you will find recipes with a heavy focus on prebiotics for their wonderful flavour, texture and health-promoting effects. I've dialled up the use of these ingredients to hit what the science deems as a reasonable amount while creating balanced recipes you can enjoy.

Probiotics are live microbes that are beneficial to us, their 'human host'. Various strains have been suggested as potential modulators of the microbiota, opening up a role for them in therapeutics. While the science around probiotics as targeted health interventions is interesting, the simplest stuff seems to be the most effective, which is why I regard prebiotics as more important to the food and health conversation than probiotics. But this should not dissuade you from trying to use probiotic foods in your daily cooking as often as possible. Experiment with ingredients like traditionally prepared kimchi, sauerkraut and probiotic yoghurt with their lactic tang to bring another flavour sensation to meals. Use them by simply folding through salads or serving on the side of a meal as a sharp, sour pairing. Try creating your own ferments and look for unpasteurised varieties in grocery stores that are full of different strains of microbes.

Polyphenols
Probably my favourite topic of discussion is plant chemicals, also referred to as phytonutrients or phytochemicals. These are the thousands of compounds found in fruits, vegetables, nuts and seeds that go beyond vitamins and minerals. Even though they aren't considered essential micronutrients, research suggests they are incredibly important for optimising our health. Polyphenols are a special type of plant chemical found in coloured plants like berries, cacao and squash, but they are also found in abundance in drinks like green tea and coffee.

Due to their antioxidant and anti-inflammatory activity that protects our cells from damage, we have long understood that a diet high in polyphenols has health-protective effects. Recent data shows how this may also be related to the positive effect polyphenols have on our gut microbes. Most polyphenols travel through the digestive tract into the large intestine without being degraded, where they fight off harmful bacteria, allowing your beneficial bugs to flourish and reduce intestinal inflammation. In addition, polyphenols enhance the function of microbes that nourish your gut cells and demonstrate the ability to increase a bacteria called *Akkermansia muciniphila*. This is of particular interest to many of us because higher amounts of this bacteria in the gut have been associated with a lower weight and lower likelihood of metabolic problems like type 2 diabetes.

When it comes to polyphenols, the more the better. They are found to be the highest in herbs and spices. Clove, star anise, oregano, sage and rosemary top the list for the most polyphenols by weight, along with curry spices, turmeric and cinnamon not far behind. This is your invitation to explore as many different cuisines as possible, in the knowledge that collecting a variety of herbs and spices along the way will benefit your health immeasurably. For that reason, you will find recipes in this book inspired by cuisines with a long tradition of pairing health-promoting ingredients: Sri Lankan dishes with curry leaves and pepper, alongside Middle Eastern-inspired meals with an abundance of soft herbs, and Asian-style broths infused with the aromatic warmth of star anise. Invest in a spice cupboard because these rich flavours are key to looking after your body and bugs, while creating wonderful, exciting food.

As well as spices, polyphenols are found in cherries, plums, blueberries, blackcurrants and other dark-coloured fruits. They are also present in nuts and seeds, such as pecans, hazelnuts and flaxseeds. You will spot these ingredients across my recipes for the same reason: intense flavour and functional benefits.

Plants

The reality is, we eat a combination of foods at each meal and by focusing on the singular characteristics of our ingredients, we risk losing sight of an important aspect of our diet. Food synergy. While it's fascinating to understand the mechanisms behind how individual foods can exert health-promoting effects, it's equally important to examine what 'blends' of ingredients are associated with health and longevity.

Combinations of foods appear to have additive effects, and the nutrients from different fruits and vegetables when consumed together interact with each other to further enhance their health-promoting properties. For example, animal studies have shown that a blend of polyphenol-rich foods, such as broccoli, apples and berries, have enhanced positive effects on the gut compared to the impact of singular foods. In addition, studies have shown that the number of unique plants that we consume on a weekly basis is associated with a healthier microbial population. In fact, just 30 different plants a week is enough diversity in the diet to achieve these remarkable health benefits. Patterns of eating that typically contain a diverse range and combination of plants in the diet, like 100% wholefood, plant-based diets and Mediterranean diets, are reflective of the potential additive effects from nutrient interactions on our gut. These diets universally demonstrate better microbe profiles, lower intestinal inflammation and overall better health.

Through the lens of gut health, we can understand why we see these results in observational research. Several studies have shown that an increase in wholefood plant intake leads to an increase in the diversity and function of your gut microbes. More plants in the daily diet also shifts the pattern towards beneficial microbes like *bifidobacteria* and *lactobacilli* and away from harmful bacteria, such as *enterococcus*. Plants like whole nuts and seeds contain a number of bioactive ingredients, such as phytosterols and vitamin E. When combined with other fibre- and nutrient-rich ingredients like lentils and beans, they further protect and bolster your microbes' function.

Unequivocally, all roads lead to a plant-focused diet. The more plants in a diet, better health outcomes are observed in large population studies that span different countries and cultures. There is nothing more certain about nutritional medicine and, despite how sensational this may sound, the evidence does not lie. A plant-focused diet lowers the risk of cancer, heart disease, kidney disease, diabetes and even mental health conditions.

Eating more plants is certainly the way forward. I am, and have always been, predominantly plant-based, and 'plant-focused' is my mantra. I welcome the trend towards flexitarian and even fully plant-based eating, especially as it encourages people to be more conscious about their plates. However, I'm of the opinion that the optimal human diet still includes some animal products, but I see these inclusions as once or twice a week luxuries, rather than daily staples. For this reason, you will find some recipes in this book that use quality fish and poultry.

Putting all this together, any strategy for improving health has to be centred around assisting our microbes, so they happily slave away at our service 7 days a week without taking any vacations. Consistently eating a diverse range of fruits, vegetables, nuts and seeds, including more prebiotics and polyphenol-rich foods, is critical to keeping microbes happy and in balance. But far from what many health-food outlets will tell you, the key lies in humble wholefoods that are usually accessible for most of us. I see the growing popularity of foods that support our microbes as a return to traditional ways of eating that were developed by our ancestors. It's a way of eating that modern science determines has the greatest concordance with gut microbial health. And hopefully my recipes will convince you that it's also a delicious way to do so.

Look at this advice through the lens of incredible, diverse foods that will take you on a journey through regional cuisines and tell a story of tradition, rather than just a collection of ingredients you ought to include in your diet because the doctor said so.

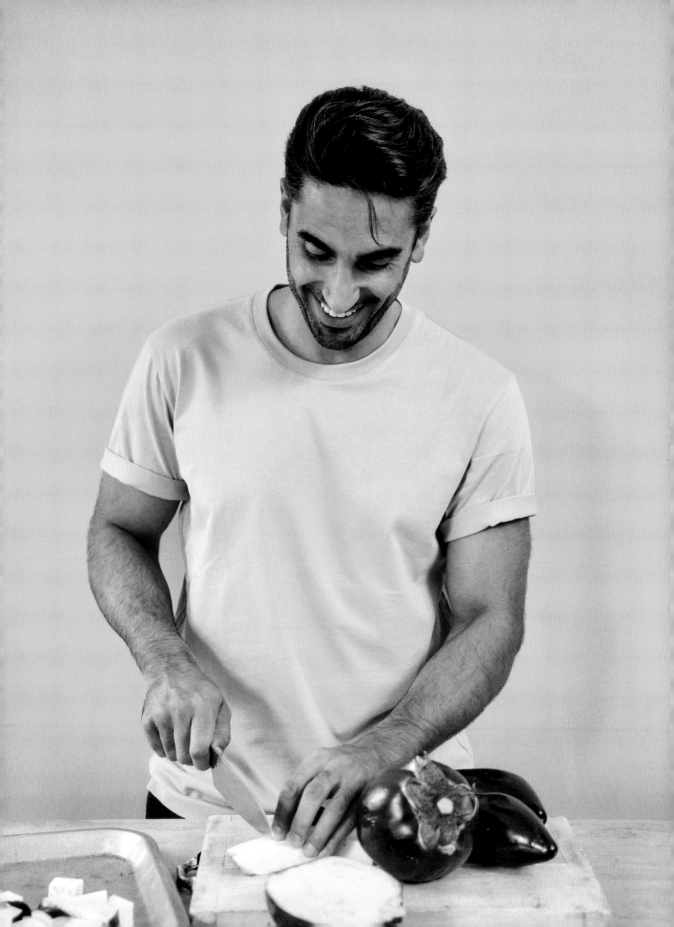

WHAT MAKES A DOCTOR'S KITCHEN RECIPE?

Throughout my media work, podcasts, books and even my TEDx talk, I've promoted the central idea that food should be considered a form of medicine to treat and prevent ill health. It's incredibly naïve to regard the realm of medicine as just the prescription of drugs or surgical interventions. As critical as those might be, medicine is so much more.

Food is exceptionally special. Through diet, we can create a healthier, more proactive population empowered to look after their own health and wellbeing. However, the concept of 'food as medicine' is commonly misrepresented by charlatans who sell supplements and diets as cure-alls and replacements for pharmaceuticals. In addition, there is a stubborn contingent of medical practitioners who leave the responsibility of diet and lifestyle advice to dieticians and health coaches, which I believe is a squandered opportunity. We can utilise food as one of the most effective tools to prevent disease and promote health; and we should be better training our clinicians to do so.

The utility of food in medicine in all its various applications is beyond the scope of this book. Instead, let me introduce you to the spectrum of food as medicine, where diet can be used to manage health as preventative medicine, supportive medicine and, in a minority of circumstances, as the core treatment.

Preventative
We already have enough real-world data to demonstrate that a diet made up of wholefoods, quality fats and a diverse range of plants results in better health outcomes across the board. Better brain health, heart health, kidney function, lower risks of cancer, lower risks of type 2 diabetes, and more. No comparable pharmaceutical offers the same preventative benefits. This is the foundation of the food-as-medicine philosophy.

Supportive
Diet plays a pivotal role in the management of patients in many different areas of medicine - from supporting recovery after a surgical procedure, maintaining physical resilience during cancer therapy to even preventing muscle mass loss in elderly

patients. As a support tool, diet can enhance performance, improve recovery and increase longevity. Alongside our suite of treatments, it deserves more attention and research funding.

Treatment

On my podcast, I've discussed the wide application of nutritional medicine at length and where, in a few circumstances, diet can be the main treatment. For example, a number of trials show low-carbohydrate diets are game changing for type 2 diabetes patients, even demonstrating remission of the disease in some. We've long known about the successful use of ketogenic diets in treating refractory epilepsy in childhood, as well as certain short-term, low FODMAP diets for irritable bowel syndrome.

Established institutions are leaning into the idea of food as medicine. The National Institute of Health in the US recently commissioned research into the concept of 'prescription meals'. In addition, they funded investigation into personalised nutrition protocols using genetic information, stool testing, metabolic parameters and wearable data.

As promising as this future sounds, I truly believe mainstream dietary advice will not veer far from the principles we already understand and can explain. The objectives will be to create consistent habits and foster a salutogenic environment where healthy options are the default. With that in mind, let's nail the basics of eating well every day, keeping it simple and achievable.

What makes these Doctor's Kitchen recipes different?

The recipes in this book are focused on the preventative medicinal benefits of food. To reinforce gut health, to lower inflammatory burden, to enhance detoxification and to support normal metabolism. These attributes are what make a Doctor's Kitchen recipe different from the norm.

The core principles on which each recipe is formulated have remained consistent throughout the years because the fundamental science has not drastically changed, despite what you might have read in sensationalist headlines. The five key attributes woven through each recipe continue to be: minimally processed wholefoods, plenty of fibre types, quality fats, diverse colourful ingredients and a focus on plants.

To this end, I maximise the use of wholefoods while minimising refined carbohydrates and sugar, to create easy meals packed with the nutrition provided by nature. To increase diversity,

I introduce as many colourful ingredients as possible. I use nuts and seeds for their distinct flavour and texture, as well as their rich mineral content and anti-inflammatory benefits. Humble high-fibre ingredients, like peas, beans and lentils, regularly take the lead role in my meals. Associated with better cardiovascular health, these complex nutritional powerhouses are critical to creating a nutritionally complete, satiating meal that feeds our microbiota with the food they require to thrive.

Research has shown that the ideal fruit and vegetable consumption is in excess of 800g per day, equivalent to 10 portions by UK standards. Therefore, every one of my recipes is formulated to contain at least three portions of vegetables, fruit, nuts or seeds to give you an ample dose of prebiotics, phytochemicals, protein, fibres and other essential nutrients. Enjoy three of my meals each day and you will easily reach what the science determines to be the optimal intake of nutrient-rich foods that can protect and enhance your wellbeing.

Studies also suggest consuming as much plant variety as possible. Eating over 30 different plants a week is associated with health benefits and a better functioning gut population. It's another reason why I try to incorporate a variety of plants, herbs and spices in each recipe. You will effortlessly get to 30 different plants in just one day of eating my recipes. You can rest assured that the recipes in this book are created with the science of food as medicine in mind, while taking you on a journey of flavour and colour to make them exciting and aspirational, yet at the same time achievable.

Making this achievable

We live in a pill-for-every-ill culture. The idea of a collection of 'superfoods' to rid us of all ailments is an attractive yet fanciful one. However, in the same way lifting a dumbbell once a week isn't going to make you the next rippling Mr Universe, having a teaspoon of berry powder in your smoothie a couple of times a week is a drop in the ocean when it comes to the health benefits of eating well. We have to consistently eat in a way that allows the benefits to accumulate. Once we appreciate this and rise to the challenge of diet being something we commit to for the long term, we can make a concerted effort to create this reality.

Regularly eating a colourful, diverse diet is essential. These ingredients compound and work synergistically, and so creating a habit of eating daily in this way is key. In addition to making these recipes balanced from a nutritional perspective, they must be easy to make and enjoy day after day. With my knowledge of nutrition, I translate these healthful foods into meals that taste incredible and do not break the 'time bank'.

Conversely, the opposite is also true. Enjoying the odd indulgent meal with as much butter as there is potato in a silky mash served with sugary, glazed root vegetables to accompany a duck roasted in its own fat and five-spice blend is not going to tip your risk factor towards ill health. But make this a daily or even weekly indulgence and we would need to work on it.

In a spirit of honesty, you do not have to (and nor should you) rely solely on recipes to meet your daily nutritional needs. 'Non-recipe' meals constitute much of what I eat every day. Sometimes that is a bowl of short-grain brown rice, a handful of seasonal leaves, some cooked beans and a few nuts, paired with an extra virgin olive oil dressing. In minutes I have a lip-smacking, satisfying meal. That's how I action my nutrition principles on a daily basis… which frankly works! When I was a junior doctor with zero time, I wasn't making curry pastes, pan-frying seabass, creating dark roux stews or anything else of that nature. But I was eating flavourful meals because of a few hacks learnt from my mother, foodie friends, tv chefs I watched every week and – now – social media. A world of flavour is at your fingertips.

What is extra special about this book is that I reached out to my community online to test and refine the recipes before finalising them for each chapter. With the help of over a thousand volunteers from across the globe, each recipe was tested on average over ten times, assessing the simplicity, accessibility, flavour, timing, reproducibility and, of course, accuracy. I read every single in-depth review and used this incredible – and sometimes critical! – feedback to refine the methods and whittle down the equipment needed to make these wonderful health-promoting dishes. They've been tested in kitchens from around the world, from Canada to Kathmandu, and Adelaide to rural France! You can be assured that these recipes are both accessible and easy to recreate whenever you want them.

While the nutritional science is complex, the solutions are simple. I put it to you, the reader, that the answer to our overburdened health system does not lie in a single perfectly created health food, but rather in eating consistently well every day. As you'll learn about in the next chapter, flavourful, delicious food that you believe is having a positive effect on your body is just as important as the nutritional content.

THE TASTE
OF HEALTH

As you flick through the pages of recipes, my objective is to make you forget that you're eating from a 'healthy' cookbook and give you the impression that you're eating for flavour and indulgence. There is a reason for this. Food is not just a collection of ingredients for physical nourishment; it's just as important that you emotionally connect with your food and enjoy what you eat. This deeper connection with food that most 'healthy eating' or 'diet' cookbooks forget, is fundamental to a way of consistently eating well for life. It's not just that healthy food *can* taste delicious, it's that it *should* taste delicious.

To be fully nourished, food must be an immersive experience that awakens our taste senses and delivers a near spiritual experience that sustains more than just our bodies. Taking pleasure from what you eat is a must. Part of my job as a doctor is to show you what to eat, but as a home cook it's also to ensure you enjoy both the cooking and the tasting experience.

I agree this esoteric way of looking at food might seem contrived, but there is some science behind it. Sensory information about food is coming from receptors in the body – your eyes, ears, nose and mouth – which gets processed in the primary sensory cortices of the brain. If you eat a subjectively delicious-tasting meal, these stimuli coalesce to create a positive experience that rewards your behaviour and encourages repetition. We get the opportunity to have rewarding experiences like these two or three times a day, which over time creates a habit.

To create a healthy-eating habit, whereby the choice of foods that serve the function of your body becomes subjectively desirable and automatic, we must strive to make this a positive experience sensorily and physically. This is to say, we can't rely on willpower alone to want to eat green vegetables, legumes and fruit just because we know they're 'good for us'. The consumption of these foods has to be a pleasurable experience, which is why my recipes intertwine flavour and function.

Pleasure research shows our basic motivation for food, sex and social interaction is fundamental to our survival and takes precedence over other aspects of our existence. Food is critical to survival, so we are hardwired to love it. It's a route to pleasure and essential for wellbeing, as is the nutritive content of food.

Often overlooked, our mindset about eating healthy foods has a significant impact on our ability to form a habit. There is an assumption that if people understand the health benefits of food or other lifestyle behaviours, they naturally align themselves to these choices. But behavioural psychology tells us otherwise. Our thoughts, beliefs and expectations of pleasurable food experiences are stronger drivers for engaging in that behaviour.

If we create anticipation by describing food or drink as pleasurable, there is heightened activity in the medial orbital frontal cortex, the pleasure centre of the brain. Studies have demonstrated that describing food according to its health attributes, such as calorie count or cholesterol benefits, is less likely to create a habit of eating well compared to describing how tasty, exciting and delicious the food is.

Despite our best intentions, most of us instinctively prioritise tastiness over healthiness when choosing what to eat, especially when time-poor and lacking in sleep. Many people believe that healthy foods are not enjoyable or satisfying, but research shows that the same foods can be experienced as more delicious depending on how they are described. Real-world studies show that labelling vegetables with indulgent descriptors, like 'zingy carrots' or 'crispy broccoli' significantly increases the number of people choosing vegetables and the total amount consumed compared with basic or healthy descriptions, despite no change in the actual product.

In other words, people are far more likely to engage in a healthy way of eating if you focus on the pleasurable characteristics of food first, rather than the health benefits. This fact chimes well with my own experience. As someone who has sat across from many patients trying to motivate a healthier-eating habit, I've always found the best way to entice people is to create an exciting promise, focusing on the appealing qualities of food that suit their tastes, preferences and norms. It's why I have included a section on dinner parties, so healthy eating in social settings with friends, family and loved ones can be normalised rather than a healthy diet being reinforced as a punitive, solitary practice.

Regardless of where you are on your healthy-eating journey, your mindset matters. It can be influenced by your intention to

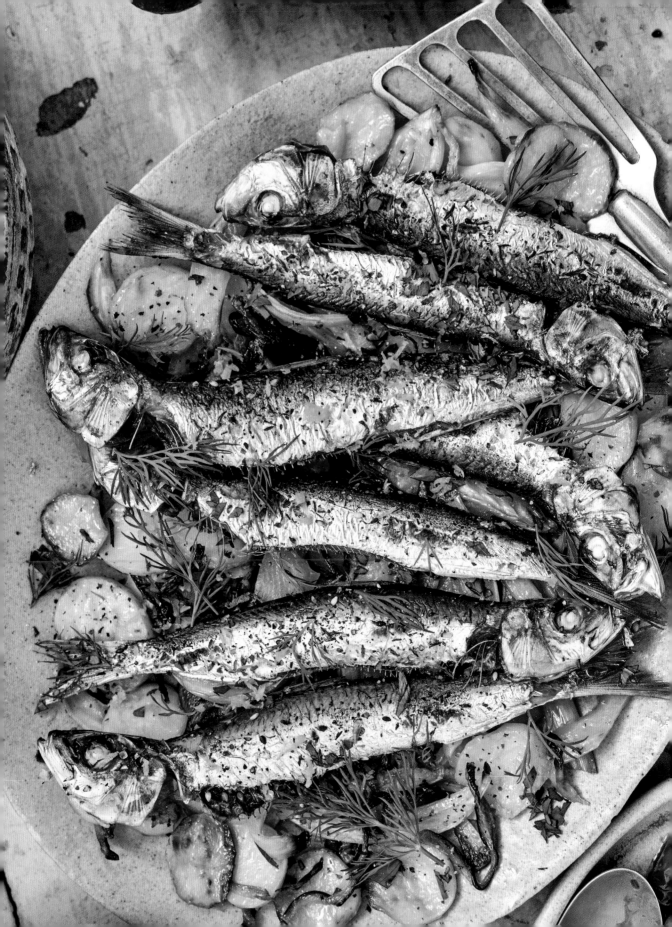

affirm and reinforce your desired behaviours across diet and other lifestyle practices, which are just as important. Believing healthy eating is enjoyable and rewarding is something I hope to convince you of in order to change your mindset for good.

From my own experience of overcoming ill health early in my life, I know it's possible to develop an affinity to foods that serve and protect you. You can cross that invisible threshold through consistency. This diet – if you want to call it that – is a way of eating that becomes automatic. My approach is far less restrictive, more adventurous and ultimately enjoyable.

There is, of course, stiff competition. The standard American diet (depressingly referred to as SAD), consisting of highly refined junk food, has been developed over decades to be palatable, pleasurable, scalable, portable and, of course, very cheap. Add billions of pounds' worth of marketing into the mix and target young people to make it seem fashionable, and no wonder it's so popular and pervasive. For a lot of people, we need to retrain our taste buds to appreciate the complexity of whole natural food, which can take months, but it's possible.

Forged by the food industry, there is also an illusion of nobody having the time or energy to cook, which is steadily dismantling the culture of home cooking. In reality, cooking is quicker, easier and far healthier for you than any delivery. I've made sure that my recipes have been formulated to be deeply practical. There is no point in creating fussy dishes that require hours of cooking time when the mission is to democratise healthy eating for everyone. This book is still a fun, foodie cookbook to be well-thumbed in kitchens across the world.

Hopefully I can show you a way of eating to be enjoyed for life. The recipes are for inspiration and demonstrate how you can eat delicious, gratifying food that fulfils emotionally as well as nutritionally. My 'flavour and function' motto represents the holistic nourishment of food, as well as its medicinal properties. Comprised of delicious, wholesome ingredients, my recipes feel like comfort eating when, in reality, they're fantastically good for your body and soul and make you feel lighter and energetic.

I want to convince you that eating to support your mental and physical health to feel fantastic *can* and *should* taste incredible. Welcome to the Doctor's Kitchen way of eating, I know it's one you're going to thoroughly enjoy. Wherever you are on your healthy-eating journey, I can make it that little bit more delicious.

HOW TO USE
THIS BOOK

There are a number of icons assigned to each recipe in this book and so, if you have particular dietary requirements, these will help you quickly find what you need. If you're looking for ways to make a dish vegetarian, vegan or gluten-free, or simply swap ingredients to use up what you already have, then check out the substitutions that I have included for many recipes too. There is a lot of variability across products, so for all substitutions, please make sure you check the packaging for allergens as needed.

Occasionally there are omissions as well as additions, where an ingredient can be skipped or added to give equally good results. As many of you will know, my recipes call for lots of spices, but these are fantastic storecupboard ingredients and will keep for at least three months. These tips and suggestions should come in super handy, plus at the back you will find a section on how to use up some of the more novel ingredients that feature in the recipes.

Each recipe has a prep time and a cook time, so you can easily plan your mealtimes. Check out the cook's index at the back for no-cook and low-cook meals, prep ahead recipes, batch cooks and one-pan dishes of which there are many to choose from!

I'm super excited for you to get stuck into this cookbook! Foodies from the UK, France, Germany, Australia, Canada, South America, India, and beyond, have all cooked these Doctor's Kitchen recipes in their homes. I reviewed their extensive feedback before refining each recipe that made it into this book. These are recipes that really work and people already absolutely love.

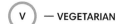 — **VEGETARIAN**

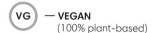 — **VEGAN**
(100% plant-based)

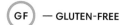 — **GLUTEN-FREE**

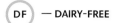 — **DAIRY-FREE**

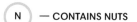 — **CONTAINS NUTS**

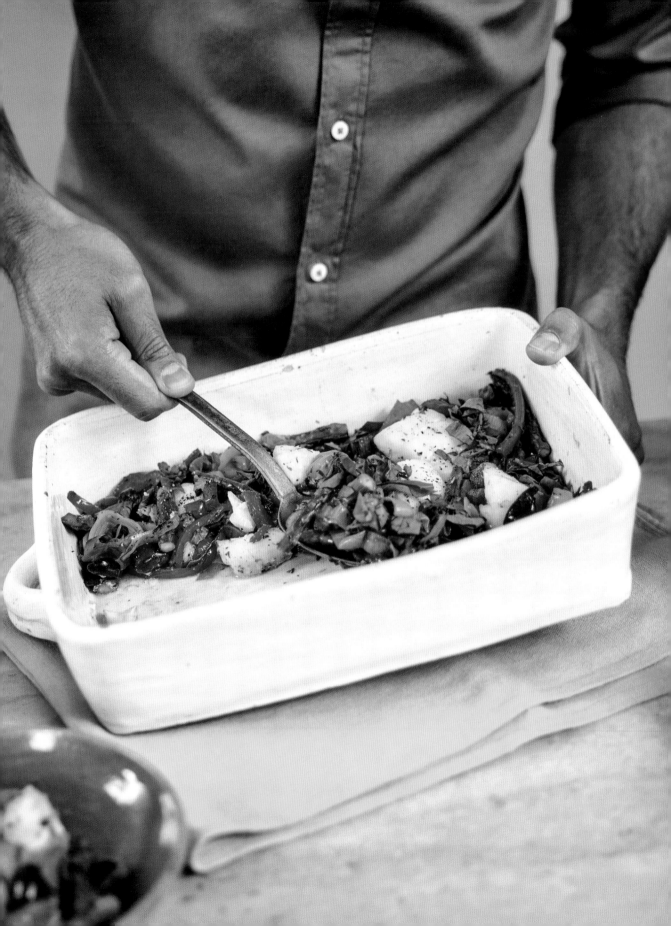

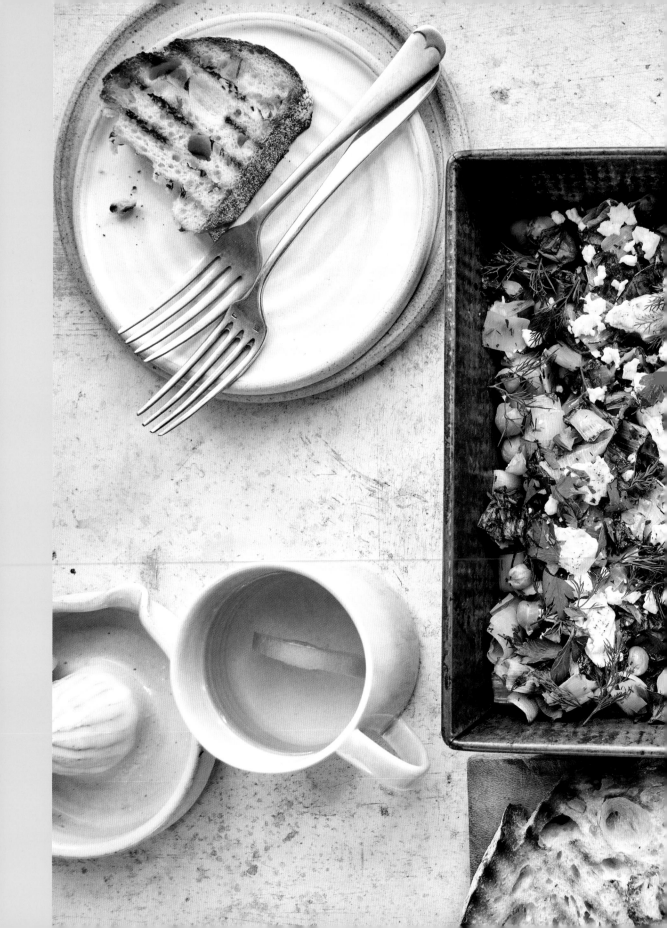

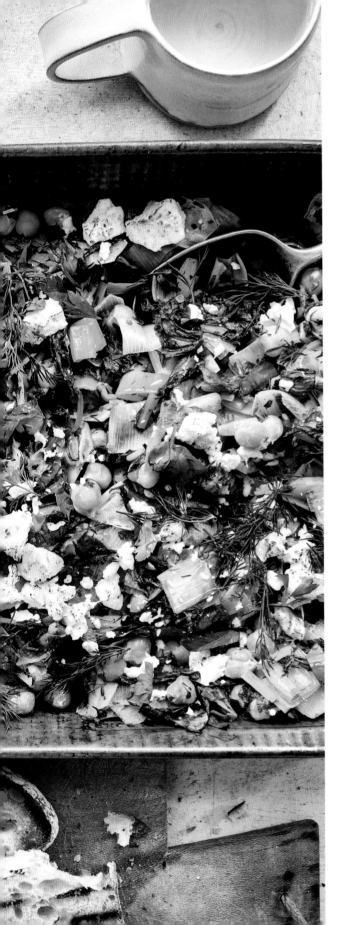

BRUNCH

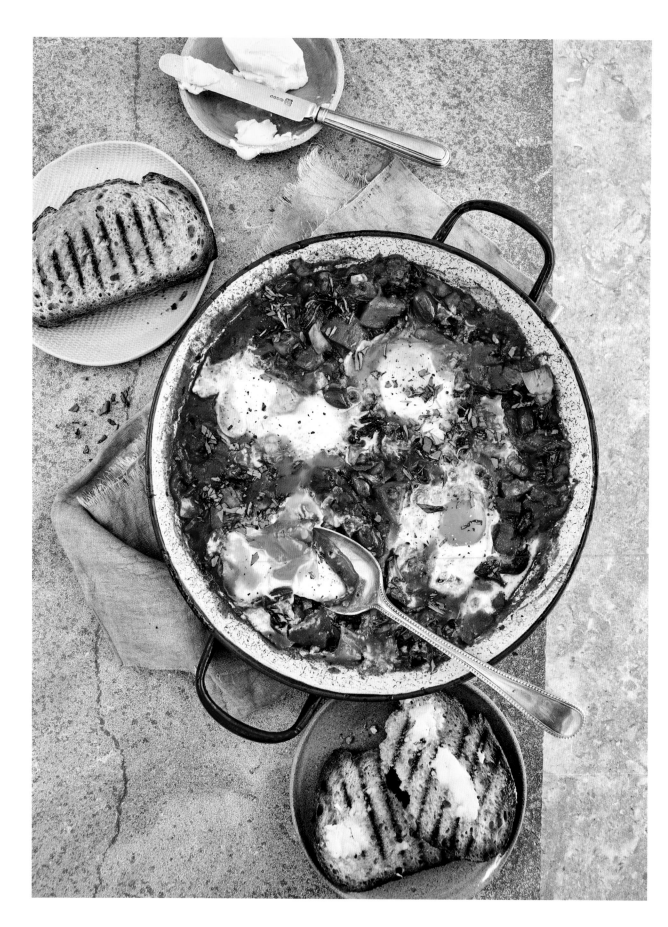

ANTIPASTI EGGS

Serves 2 generously

Prep time: 15 minutes
Cook time: 20 minutes

This Mediterranean-inspired tangy, sweet and delicious brunch dish is balanced in flavours and has multiple textures that you will love. The beautiful antipasti ingredients give a glorious sharp flavour which is mellowed by the sweetness of the soft herbs and tomatoes.

1 tbsp extra virgin olive oil

200g rainbow chard, stalks chopped, leaves shredded

160g artichokes in brine, drained and roughly chopped

3 large roasted red peppers (180g), from a jar, drained and roughly chopped

60g walnuts, crumbled

30g pitted kalamata olives

30g tomato purée

200g passata

1 tsp dried oregano

1 tsp smoked paprika (optional)

4 medium eggs

Small bunch of tarragon, leaves roughly chopped

Sourdough toast or **gluten-free bread slices**, to serve

Heat the oil in a shallow flameproof casserole that has a lid over a medium-high heat.

Add the chard stalks, artichokes, peppers, walnuts and olives and fry for 3 to 4 minutes until the chard stalks have softened.

Lower the heat to medium, stir in the tomato purée, fry for 1 minute, then add the passata, oregano and paprika, if using. Bring to a simmer, then cover and cook for 5 minutes.

Stir in the chard leaves, put the lid back on the casserole and cook for 2 to 3 minutes until wilted, then check the seasoning.

Use the back of a spoon or a ladle to make 4 hollows in the mixture, then crack an egg into each. Cover with the lid and cook for 4 to 5 minutes until the egg whites are set and the yolks are still runny.

Scatter over the chopped tarragon and serve straight away with buttered sourdough toast.

Substitutions

Rainbow chard: spinach or regular chard

Jarred roasted peppers: finely chopped fresh red pepper

Tarragon: dried tarragon or extra oregano to finish

POACHED EGGS & LEMON GREENS WITH HAZELNUT DUKKAH

Serves 2

Prep time: 10 minutes
Cook time: 15 minutes

A fresh dukkah in the making, with the scent of the coriander seeds gently toasting away in the pan, is the signal for the weekend in my mind. The earthy spices and nuts in this Middle Eastern blend are made infinitely better when you prepare it from scratch. Tossed through seasonal greens, a dash of good olive oil and lemon is all you need for a perfectly balanced start to the day.

4 medium eggs

Sourdough toast or **gluten-free bread slices**, to serve

For the hazelnut dukkah

1 tbsp coriander seeds

1 tbsp sesame seeds

2 tsp cumin seeds

2 tsp fennel seeds

60g roasted chopped hazelnuts

For the lemon greens

2 tbsp extra virgin olive oil

200g rainbow chard, roughly chopped

200g kale, stems removed, roughly chopped

2 garlic cloves, grated

Pared zest and juice of 1 lemon, 3 strips of zest pared using a swivel peeler

For the dukkah, tip all the seeds into a dry frying pan, set over a medium heat and toast for 2 to 3 minutes, until fragrant. Tip into a pestle and mortar, add the hazelnuts and a pinch of salt and grind to a coarse powder.

Wipe the pan out with a piece of kitchen paper, set over a medium heat and add the oil for the lemon greens.

Add the chard and kale, sauté for 2 to 3 minutes then add the grated garlic, some seasoning, the lemon zest, and a splash of water, and cover with a lid. Steam for 3 to 4 minutes until wilted, then remove from the heat, stir in the lemon juice and check the seasoning.

Meanwhile, poach the eggs in a pan of gently simmering water for 3 to 4 minutes until the whites are set and the yolks still runny.

Pile the greens onto the toast, top with the eggs and sprinkle over the dukkah to serve.

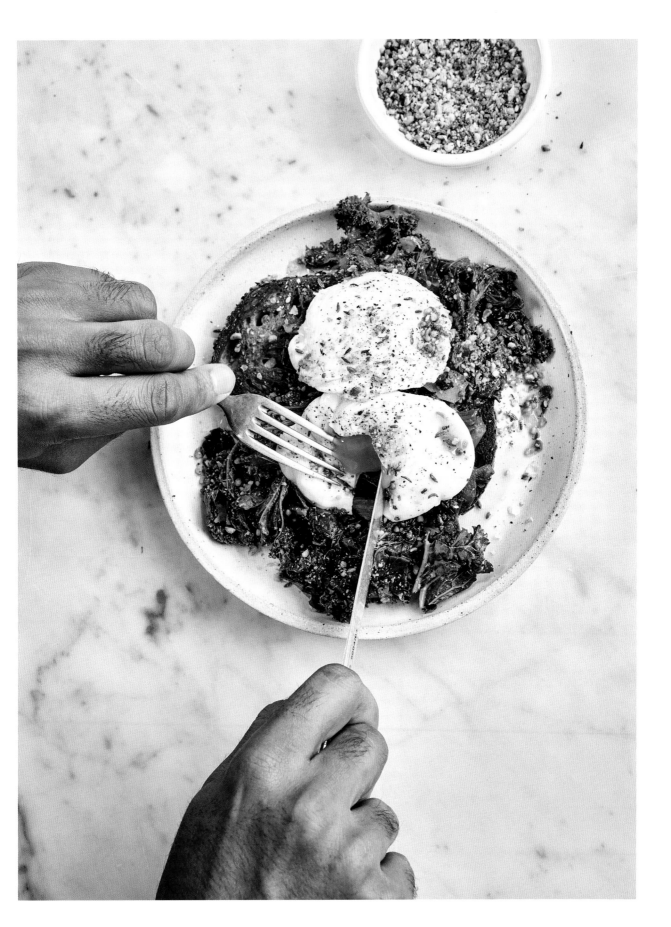

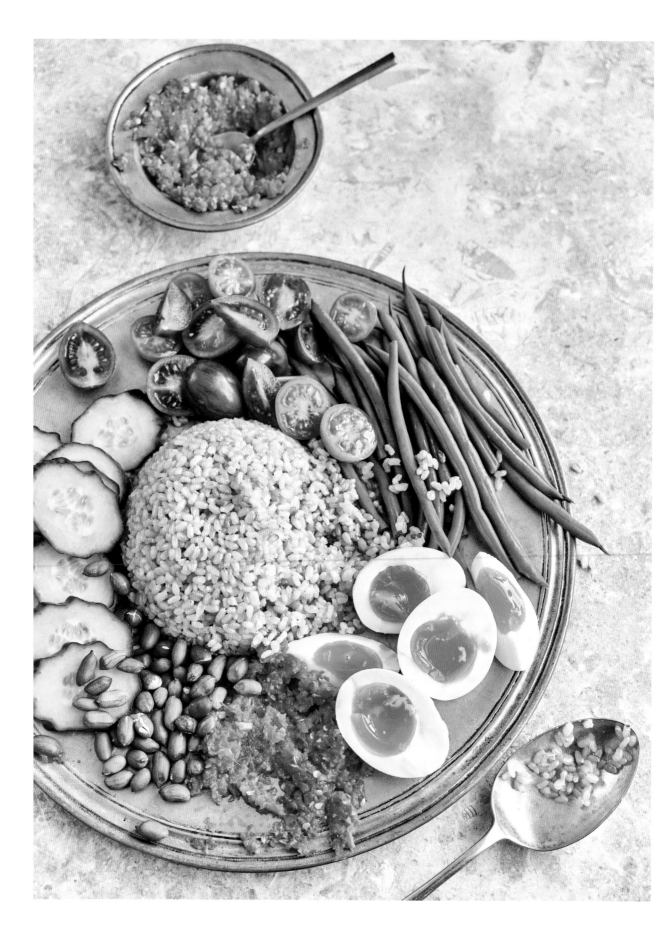

COCONUT RICE WITH SOFT-BOILED EGGS & SAMBAL

Serves 2

Prep time: 20 minutes
Cook time: 45 minutes

Inspired by a nasi lemak, the adventurous ensemble of flavours in this meal will certainly perk up your brunch options. Coconutty rice, fiery sambal and fresh green beans combine to give an amazing aroma, flavour and texture. Serve a vegetarian sambal to keep this veggie-friendly.

200g short-grain brown rice

250ml coconut milk

1 lemongrass stalk, bashed

160g green beans, trimmed

2 medium eggs

1 tbsp tamari or **light soy sauce**

1 tbsp rice vinegar

160g baby tomatoes, halved

¼ cucumber, sliced

60g skin-on roasted red peanuts

2–3 tbsp Quick Sambal (see below), to serve

Tip the rice into a flameproof casserole or wide saucepan and stir in the coconut milk with 250ml water, then add the lemongrass and a pinch of salt. Bring to the boil, then reduce the heat to a gentle simmer. Cover with a lid and cook for 30 minutes or until tender. Add the green beans to the pan for the last 5 minutes of cooking (with the lid on). Take off the heat and leave to stand for 5 minutes before serving.

Meanwhile, bring a small pan of water to the boil, add the eggs and cook for 7 minutes. Drain, then lower the eggs into a bowl of iced water and leave to cool. Peel the eggs underwater (the shells come away more easily), then drain and set aside.

Discard the lemongrass stalk, arrange the rice in the middle of a platter and pile the green beans on one side. Season with the soy sauce and rice vinegar, add the tomatoes, cucumber and peanuts to the dish. Halve the eggs and place on the platter with a large spoonful of sambal.

QUICK SAMBAL

Makes about 150g

200g red chillies, roughly chopped

2 shallots, roughly chopped

6 garlic cloves, peeled and bashed

1 lemongrass stalk, tough outer leaves removed, chopped

3 tbsp water

3 tbsp rice vinegar

1 tbsp sugar

1 tsp shrimp paste or **tamari** or **light soy sauce**

Put all the ingredients into a food processor and blend to a coarse paste. Pour into a saucepan, bring to a simmer for 10 minutes until thickened. Remove from the heat and leave to cool.

Pour into a sterilised jar, cover with a lid and keep in the fridge for up to one month. This sambal is quite fiery, so if you want to turn down the heat you can deseed half or all of the chillies.

KOREAN ONE-PAN EGGS

Serves 2

Prep time: 10 minutes
Cook time: 25 minutes

The rich, tomatoey sauce is delicious and spicy in this perfect brunch-style dish packed with vegetables. The gochujang gives a sweet heat that carries through the green vegetables and eggs. This pairs well with some short-grain brown rice.

2 tbsp sesame oil

100g spring onions, finely chopped

100g kimchi

2 tbsp gochujang

1 tbsp doenjang or white miso paste

1 tbsp tomato purée

200g Chinese leaf cabbage, finely chopped

1 x 400g can chopped tomatoes

4 medium eggs

2 tsp toasted sesame seeds

2 sheets of toasted nori, quartered, to serve

Heat the oil in a flameproof casserole or sauté pan that has a lid over a medium heat. Add the spring onions, reserving some of the green parts for garnish, and fry for 2 minutes until softened. Add the kimchi and fry for a further 3 minutes until most of the liquid has evaporated.

Stir in the gochujang, doenjang and tomato purée and fry for 2 minutes; the mixture should turn a deep red colour.

Add the Chinese leaf cabbage and chopped tomatoes, bring to a simmer and cook gently for 10 minutes. Add a splash of water if the mixture sticks to the bottom of the pan too much.

Using the back of a spoon or a ladle, make 4 hollows in the sauce, crack an egg into each hollow, then cover with the lid and cook for 5 minutes until the whites are just set and the yolks are still runny.

Top with the reserved spring onion greens and the toasted sesame seeds and serve with the pieces of toasted nori.

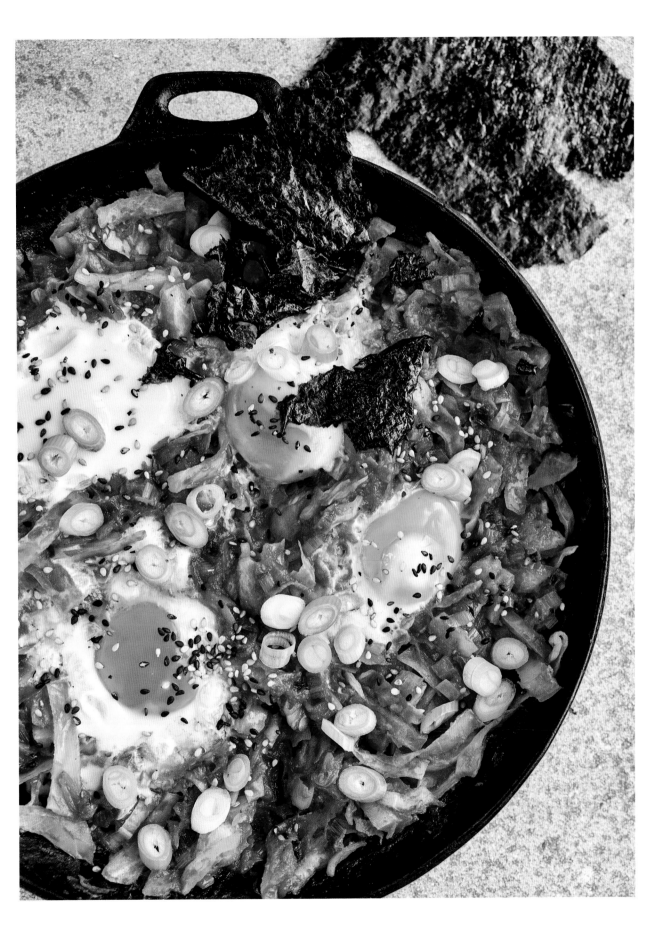

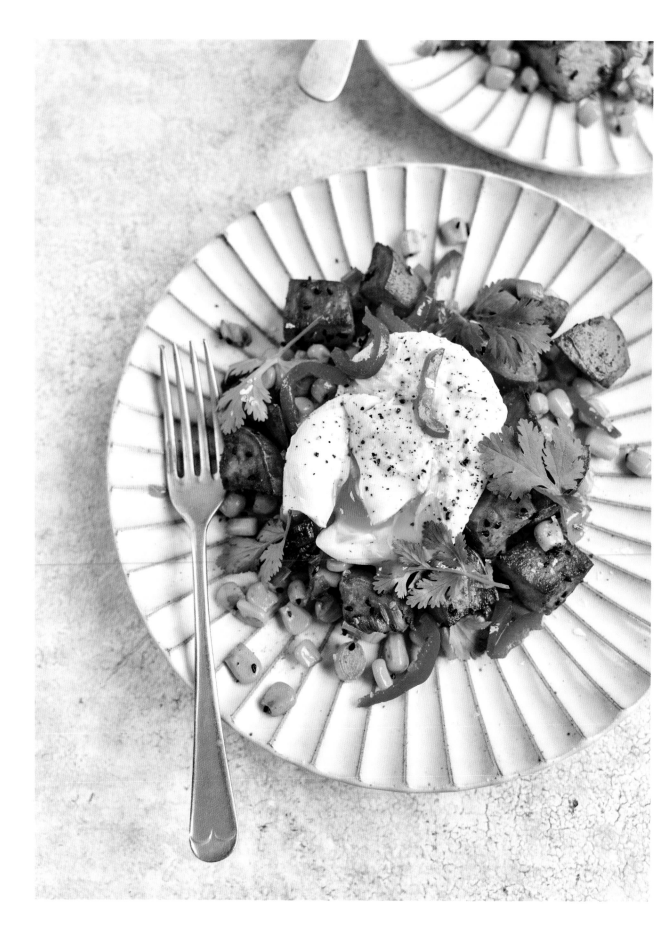

SWEET POTATO BREAKFAST HASH

Serves 2

Prep time: 15 minutes
Cook time: 20 minutes

I love this method of cooking sweet potatoes in the pan as it really concentrates those jammy notes. The leeks and sweetcorn work really well with the sweet potato to create a vibrant, flavourful dish that is a satisfying start to any weekend!

2 tbsp extra virgin olive oil

1 large sweet potato (300g), scrubbed and left unpeeled, cut into 2cm cubes

1 small leek (200g), sliced into rounds 1cm thick

1 tsp nigella seeds

½ tsp fennel seeds, roughly crushed

1 tsp sweet smoked paprika

160g drained canned or **frozen sweetcorn**

2 medium eggs

Small bunch of coriander, roughly chopped

20g red jalapeños in brine from a jar, finely sliced (optional)

Heat the oil in a shallow, flameproof, lidded casserole or frying pan over a medium heat.

Add the sweet potato, stir to coat in the oil then cover with the lid and cook gently for 10 minutes, stirring occasionally.

Add the leek, nigella seeds, fennel seeds, seasoning and paprika and cook for 6 to 7 minutes, stirring occasionally, until the leeks have cooked down and the potatoes are soft.

Stir in the sweetcorn and cook for a further 2 minutes to infuse the flavours, then take off the heat.

Meanwhile, poach the eggs in a pan of gently simmering water for 3 to 4 minutes until the whites are set and yolks are still runny.

Spoon the hash into bowls, top with the poached eggs and scatter over the coriander and sliced jalapeños, if using.

TAHINI BAKED EGGS WITH GREENS & SMOKED MACKEREL

Prep time: 10 minutes
Cook time: 20 minutes

I'm using tahini here to make a wonderfully rich sauce that creates a perfect home for the smoked fish and eggs. The lemon and fresh herbs cut through the richness of the sesame paste, and by using a lid to bake the eggs you prevent drying out the greens. This is a rich dish packed full of micronutrients and perfect for a weekend brunch.

2 tbsp extra virgin olive oil

200g Tenderstem broccoli, roughly chopped

100g baby leaf spinach, chopped (or rocket)

40g chives, chopped

150g smoked mackerel or **smoked haddock**, skin removed and broken into 3cm chunks

2 medium eggs

Toasted rye bread or **wholegrain pitta**, to serve (optional)

For the tahini sauce

60g tahini (whole or light)

2 tsp za'atar or **dukkah spice mix** (see page 32 for homemade)

Juice of 1 lemon, plus extra to serve

120ml hot water

Preheat the oven to 200°C fan.

Whisk the tahini with the spices, lemon juice and hot water until it reaches a light, yoghurt-like consistency (you may need to add more hot water) and set aside.

Heat the oil over a medium heat in a heavy-based, flameproof, lidded casserole that has a lid. Add the broccoli and a pinch of salt and cook for 3 to 4 minutes.

Add the spinach and half the chopped chives, and cook for a further minute until wilted. Stir in the fish and cook for 1 minute, then remove from the heat.

Gently stir the tahini sauce into the ingredients. Use the back of a spoon or a ladle to create 2 hollows for the eggs, then crack an egg into each. Season and cover with a lid, then slide into the oven.

Bake for 10 minutes until the egg whites are set and the yolks still runny.

Scatter over the remaining chives and serve with an extra squeeze of lemon and toasted bread or pitta for dipping, if you like.

Substitutions

Smoked mackerel or haddock: haricot beans or borlotti beans for a vegetarian alternative

Baby-leaf spinach: rocket leaves

Note

Baked eggs: omit the eggs to make it completely plant-based

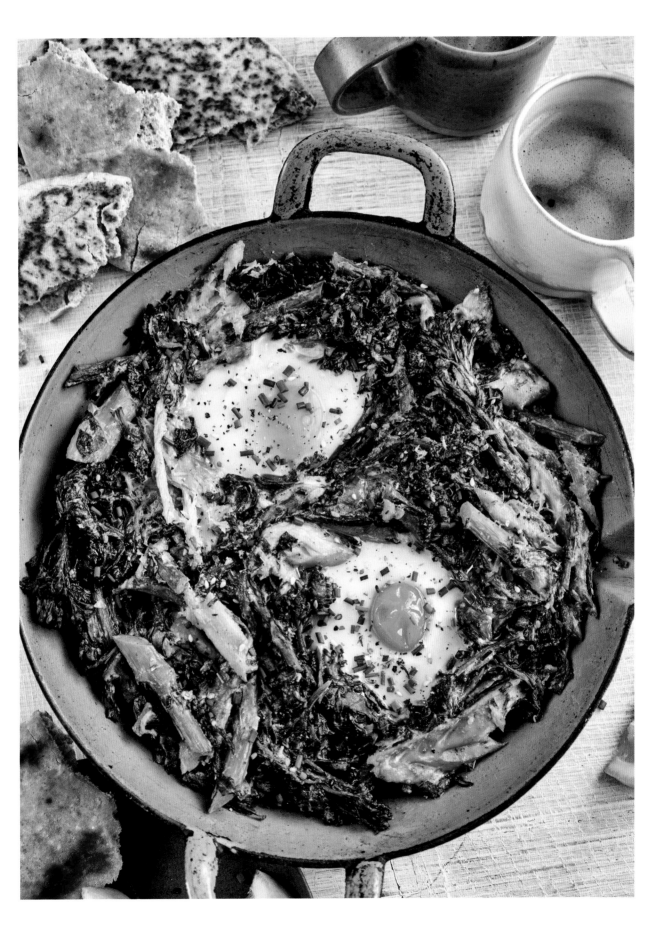

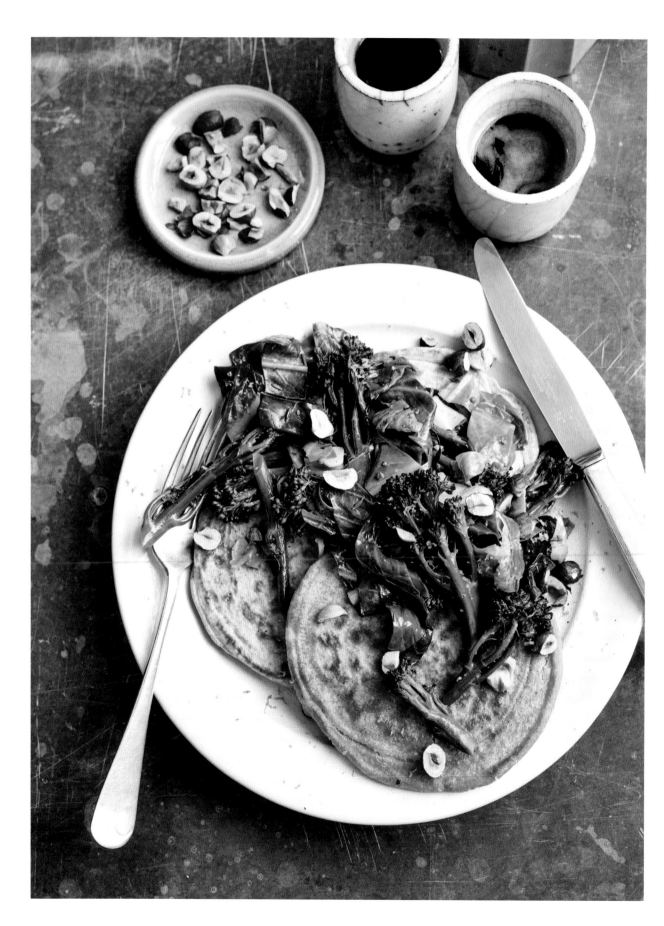

SPICY OAT PANCAKES WITH GREENS

Serves 2

Prep time: 15 minutes
Cook time: 10 minutes

One of my favourite weekend brunch dishes to make. A simple rolled oats savoury pancake with a mixture of greens and crunch from the hazelnuts. A delicious mix of quality fats, vibrant greens and pops of spice. A crowd pleaser.

For the pancakes

180g rolled oats (gluten-free, if necessary)

150ml oat milk or **almond milk**

2 large eggs

2 tsp baking powder

½ tsp salt

Pinch of chilli flakes

2 tbsp olive oil

For the greens

2 tbsp olive oil

160g Tenderstem broccoli, stems and florets separated, sliced on an angle

2 garlic cloves, sliced

1 tsp coriander seeds, crushed

1 tsp cumin seeds, crushed

½ tsp ground cinnamon

160g spring greens, roughly chopped

Pinch of chilli flakes

Finely grated zest and **juice of ½ lemon**

60g toasted chopped hazelnuts

For the pancakes, tip all the ingredients except the oil into a blender and blend to a smooth batter. Let it sit for a few minutes before making the pancakes.

Heat a little oil in a large, non-stick frying pan over a medium-high heat, then drop large spoonfuls of the batter into the pan.

Cook for 2 to 3 minutes on each side until risen and golden, then transfer to a warm plate. Continue cooking the pancakes in batches until all the batter has been used, keeping everything warm in the oven as you go.

Meanwhile, add the oil for the greens to a large sauté pan over a medium heat. Add the broccoli stems with the garlic, coriander and cumin seeds, cinnamon and a pinch of salt. Sauté for 2 to 3 minutes, then add the broccoli florets, spring greens and chilli flakes and a pinch of pepper. Cover with a lid and cook for 4 to 5 minutes until the greens have wilted and are cooked through.

Remove from the heat and stir in the lemon zest and juice, and the chopped hazelnuts.

Serve the pancakes topped with the greens.

Substitutions

Spring greens: sprout tops or cavolo nero

SWEET CORNBREAD WITH HOT HONEY, GARLICKY GREENS & TAMARIND BEANS

Serves 4 or 5 with leftover cornbread

Prep time: 30 minutes
Cook time: 50 minutes

This cornbread uses both polenta and sweetcorn, which adds wholegrain fibres and a nutty sweetness, while the hot honey takes things to another level. Pair this flavourful cornbread with garlicky greens and tamarind beans for an abundance of vegetables and happy smiles around the table.

250g drained canned sweetcorn

250g natural yoghurt

2 large eggs

1 tbsp honey

250g polenta (instant or regular)

50g plain flour

2 tsp baking powder

1 tsp salt

2 tbsp olive oil

For the hot honey

3 tbsp honey

1 tsp chilli flakes

1 tsp salt

For the garlicky greens

3 tbsp olive oil

200g white onion, diced

300g each cavolo nero and Swiss chard

5 garlic cloves, grated

For the tamarind beans

1 tbsp tamarind paste

3 tbsp tomato purée

1 tbsp honey

2 tbsp dark soy sauce

1 garlic clove, grated

1 x 400g can pinto beans, drained and rinsed

Preheat the oven to 200°C fan and set a 24cm cast-iron skillet on the middle shelf to heat.

Blend half the sweetcorn with the yoghurt, eggs and honey until smooth. Combine the polenta, flour, baking powder and salt in a bowl, then stir in the blended mixture and remaining sweetcorn.

Remove the skillet from the oven, add the olive oil and swirl it around. Pour the cornbread mixture into the skillet and smooth it out to the sides. Slide into the oven and bake for 20 minutes until risen and golden. Remove from the oven and allow to cool before serving.

Meanwhile, to make the hot honey, add the honey, chilli flakes and salt to a pan with 100ml water and bring to a gentle simmer over a medium heat until bubbling. Once it is slightly sticky and coats a spoon (about 5 to 6 minutes), drizzle over the warm cornbread.

Heat the oil for the greens in a large pan over a medium heat, add the white onion and cook for 5 to 6 minutes until softened. Meanwhile, remove the stems from the cavolo nero and finely shred the leaves. Add the greens and garlic to the pan and toss around to gently wilt. Cover with a lid and cook for about 4 to 5 minutes, then take off the heat.

Add all the ingredients for the beans, except the pinto beans, to a pan with 150ml water. Bring to a simmer for 10 minutes, then add the beans, cover with a lid and gently simmer for a further 10 minutes to infuse the beans with all the flavours.

Serve the greens and beans with wedges or slices of cornbread sprinkled with a pinch of salt.

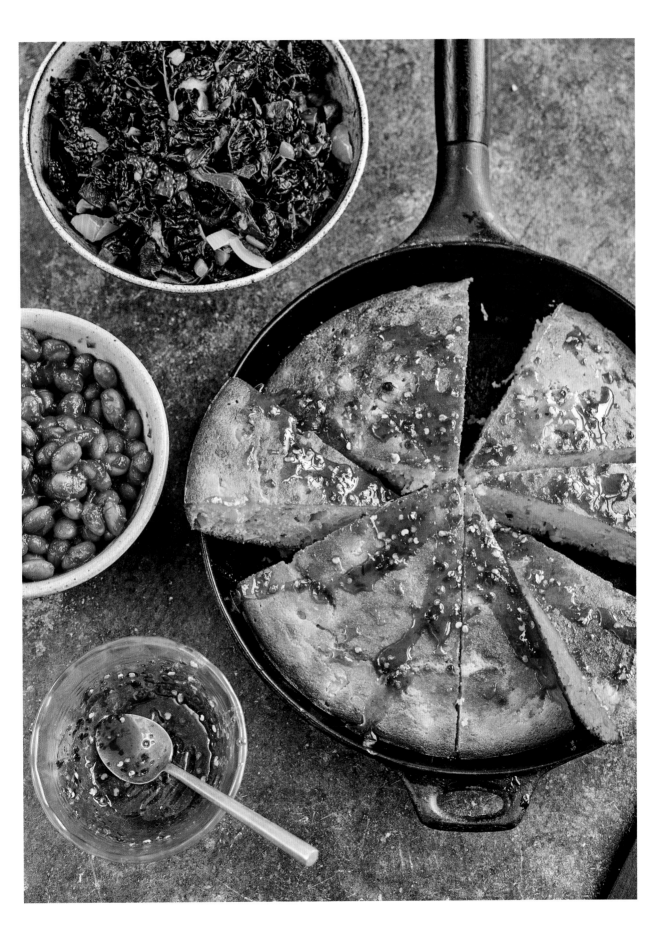

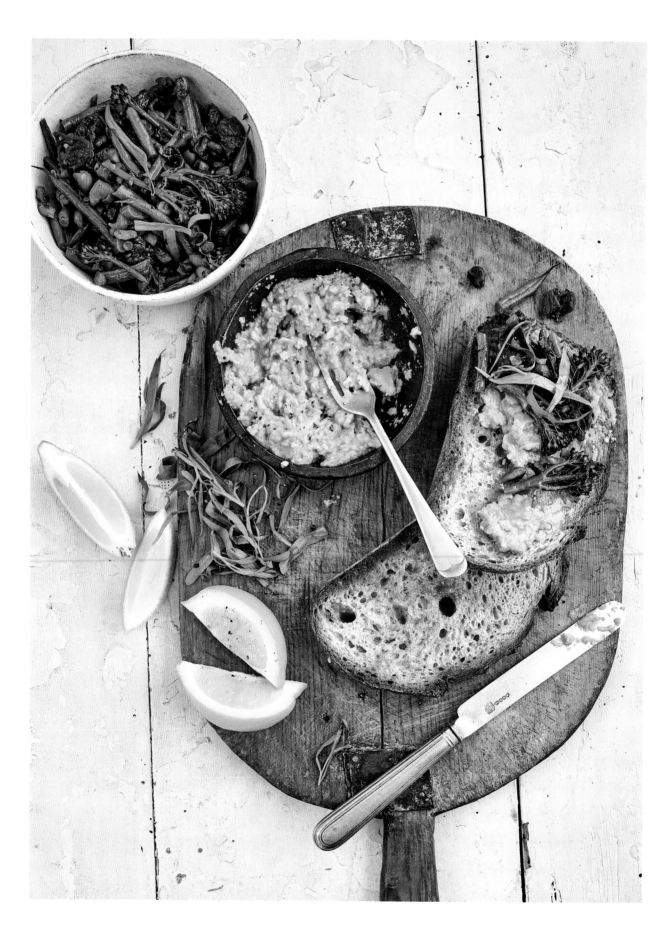

PISTACHIO GREENS & SUN-DRIED TOMATOES

Serves 2

Prep time: 15 minutes
Cook time: 10 minutes

This is a punchy-flavoured brunch dish with a great contrast of textures from the avocado and pistachios. A lovely hit of umami comes from the sun-dried tomatoes, and tarragon delivers a hint of aniseed sweetness.

2 tbsp olive oil

60g pistachios, shelled and roughly chopped

1 tsp caraway seeds

50g sun-dried tomatoes, drained and roughly chopped

160g Tenderstem broccoli, stems finely sliced, florets roughly chopped

160g green beans, roughly chopped

1 large avocado (180–200g)

Juice of ½ lemon

2 large slices of sourdough bread, toasted

Small bunch of tarragon, chopped

Heat the oil in a deep frying pan over a medium heat, add the pistachios and caraway seeds and fry for 2 minutes.

Increase the heat, add the sun-dried tomatoes, broccoli stems and beans and fry for 2 to 3 minutes.

Add the broccoli florets and a splash of water and cook for a further 2 minutes; the vegetables should be bright green and tender, with a slight crunch. Season with a pinch each of salt and pepper.

Roughly mash the avocado with the lemon juice, season, and spread on the toast. Pile the greens on top of the toast and finish with the chopped tarragon.

Substitutions

Green beans: courgette cut into batons, asparagus

Additions

Optional: add a poached egg to each plate

HERBY LEEKS WITH CHICKPEAS & CHILLI FETA

Serves 2

Prep time: 15 minutes
Cook time: 30 minutes

This gorgeous, vibrant green dish reveals how obviously good for you it is on aesthetics alone, but the complex flavours of fresh green herbs married with cumin, chilli and earthy oregano make this easy one-pan dish a complete winner all round. Make this plant-based by omitting the feta or using a nut cheese alternative.

2 tbsp extra virgin olive oil

300g leeks, sliced into half moons about 2cm thick

4 garlic cloves, sliced

2 tsp cumin seeds

2 tsp dried oregano

100g green herbs
(I use parsley and dill), stalks and leaves separated, roughly chopped

150g baby spinach, roughly chopped

1 x 400g can chickpeas, drained and rinsed

40g feta

Juice of 1 lemon

2 tbsp chilli oil (optional)

Preheat the grill to high.

Heat the olive oil in a wide, flameproof, lidded casserole over a medium heat.

Add the leeks, garlic and some seasoning, and cook gently with the lid on for 10 minutes, stirring occasionally.

Add the cumin and oregano and cook for a further 2 minutes before adding the herb stalks.

Add the spinach in batches and stir into the mixture until wilted (about 5 minutes) then add half the herb leaves, reserving the rest for garnish.

Add the chickpeas and toss through the green vegetable mixture. Crumble over the feta and transfer to the grill for a few minutes until the feta is just melted and starting to brown.

To serve, scatter over the remaining fresh herb leaves, add the lemon juice and drizzle over the chilli oil.

Substitutions

Green herbs: any mix of soft green herbs, such as coriander, tarragon and sorrel

Baby spinach: Swiss chard or rocket leaves

Leeks: fennel or chicory

Chickpeas: white beans, borlotti beans or black chickpeas

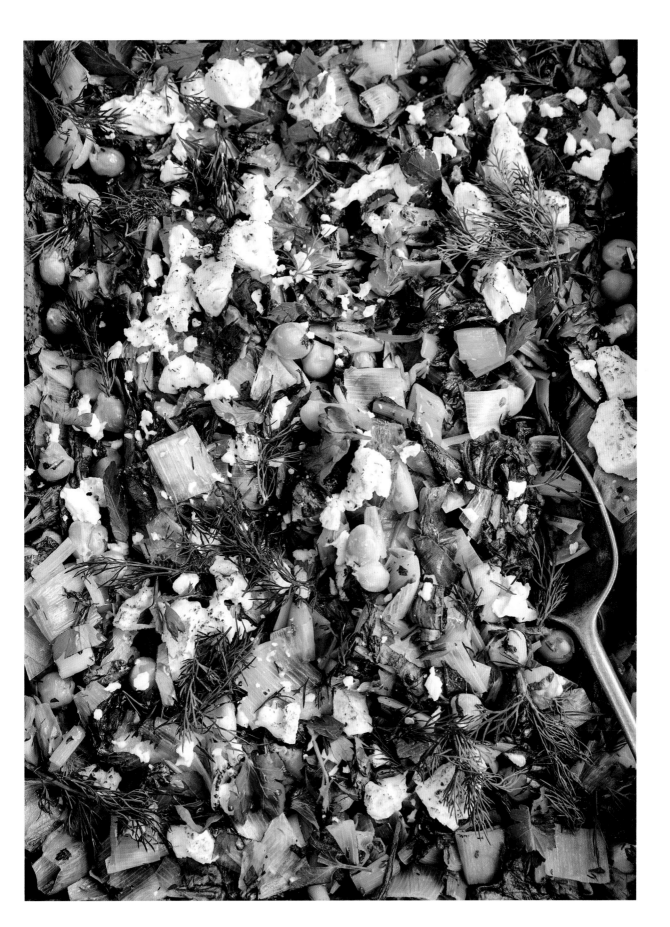

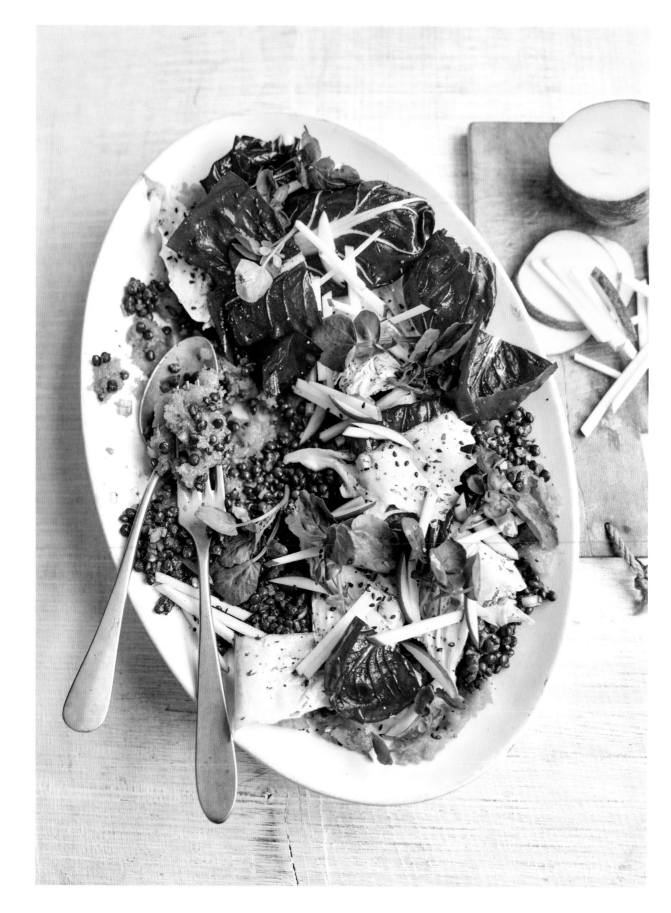

SMASHED GARLIC SQUASH WITH LENTILS & BITTER LEAVES

Serves 4

Prep time: 15 minutes
Cook time: 30 minutes

I love this platter of colour and different elements of sweetness and bitterness that come together beautifully. The dish is rich in polyphenols as well as specialised fibres from the chicory, lentils and garlic.

2 tbsp olive oil

1 tbsp white miso paste

6–8 garlic cloves, grated

1 large butternut squash, peeled, seeded and cut into 2cm cubes (800g prepped weight)

250g cooked Puy lentils

200g red chicory or radicchio leaves, roughly chopped

100g watercress, roughly torn

2 small red apples (320g), cored and cut into thin matchsticks or small dice

2 tsp black or white sesame seeds

For the dressing

3 tbsp extra virgin olive oil

2 tbsp red wine vinegar

Pinch of chilli flakes

1 small shallot (50g), finely diced

Preheat the oven to 200ºC fan. Put a roasting tin in the oven for a few minutes to heat up.

Pour the olive oil and miso paste into the roasting tin, stir in the grated garlic and then add the squash. Thoroughly mix everything so the squash pieces are evenly coated, then roast in the oven for 30 minutes, giving it all a good stir and shake a few times during cooking.

Meanwhile, whisk all the ingredients for the dressing together in a large bowl, seasoning with a pinch each of salt and pepper, then set aside.

Once the squash is soft, remove it from the oven and use a potato masher or fork to roughly mash. Spread the smashed squash over a serving platter.

Add the lentils and red leaves to the bowl of dressing, toss to coat then mound on top of the smashed squash. Scatter the watercress and apple over the platter and then sprinkle the sesame seeds on top before serving.

KOREAN PANCAKES (YACHAEJEON)

Serves 2

Prep time: 20 minutes
Cook time: 20 minutes

I love making these light, crisp vegetable pancakes as an interesting brunch dish for friends – who can help with the prep – or even a delicious snack. It's also a great way to get kids involved in the cooking process, and asking them to identify which vegetables are in the batter. The dipping sauce is simple, but perfect for these crispy morsels.

200g sweet potato, scrubbed and left unpeeled, cut into thin matchsticks or coarsely grated

160g parsnip, scrubbed and left unpeeled, cut into thin matchsticks or coarsely grated

120g gluten-free plain flour

Pinch of chilli flakes

100g spring onions, halved lengthways and cut into thin matchsticks

50g radishes, thinly sliced

Bunch of chives, roughly chopped

4 tbsp olive oil

50g kimchi, to serve

For the dipping sauce

2 tbsp tamari or **soy sauce**

1 tbsp rice vinegar

1 tsp toasted sesame seeds

Pinch of chilli flakes

Note

Gluten-free plain flour gives a far crisper exterior than wheat flour.

Put the sweet potato and parsnip matchsticks into a large bowl, add a generous pinch of salt and massage for a couple of minutes until the vegetables soften. (If you've grated them, squeeze out the excess water, dry well with kitchen paper, add the salt and omit the massaging step.)

Add the flour, chilli flakes and some freshly ground black pepper with 150ml water. Mix with your hands until the vegetables are all coated in a smooth batter.

Add the spring onions, radishes and chives and mix thoroughly, making sure all the vegetables are lightly coated in the batter.

Heat 1 tbsp of the oil in a large non-stick frying pan over a medium-low heat. Add a large spoonful of the vegetable mixture then press everything out into an even layer, about 1cm thick, using a spatula. Cook gently for 6 to 7 minutes until the underside is crisp and golden. If your pan is big enough, you can cook 2 or 3 pancakes at a time with a little extra oil.

Using a spatula, gently flip the pancake. Add a drizzle of extra olive oil to the pan and cook on the other side for a further 6 to 7 minutes, until crisp and golden.

Flip the pancake again, giving each side a further 2 to 3 minutes to cook the vegetables through and crisp up.

Meanwhile, mix the ingredients for the dipping sauce in a bowl. Slide the pancake onto a board, cut into wedges and serve with the dipping sauce and kimchi.

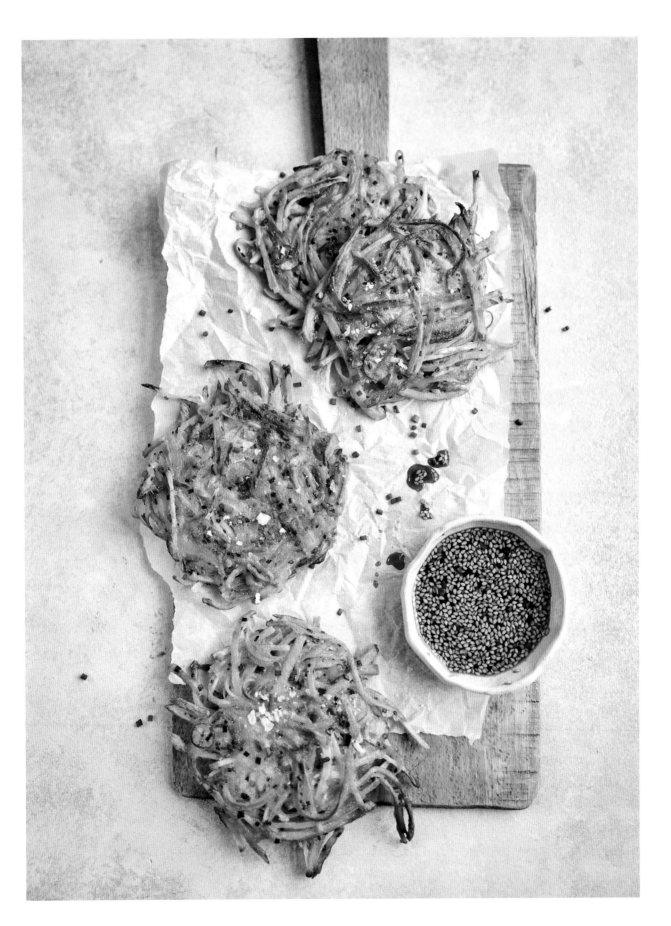

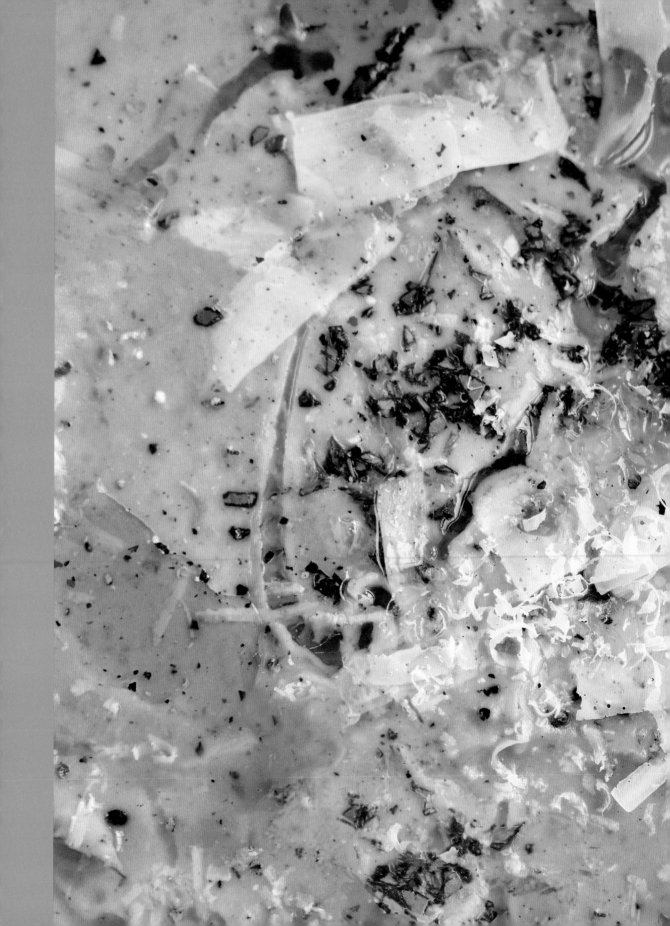

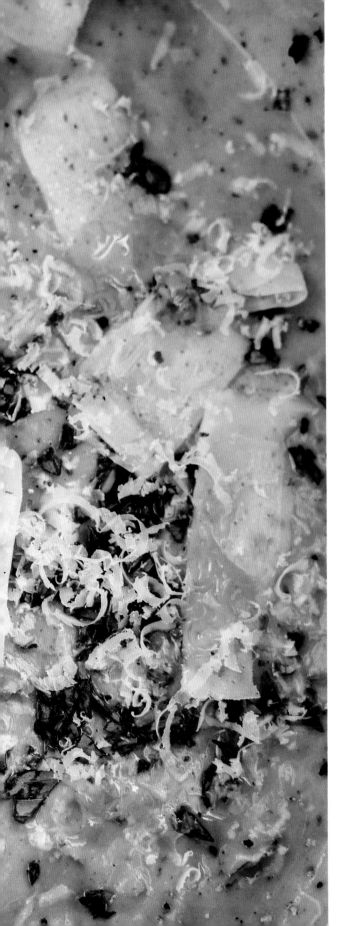

SOUPS
& BROTHS

ALMOND SALMOREJO

Serves 2

Prep time: 15 minutes, plus chilling
Cook time: 5 minutes

A cooling summery Spanish staple packed with quality fats from the almonds, beautiful sweet tomatoes and roasted peppers with hits of acidity from the vinegar and garlic. Preparing the almonds and tomatoes takes a little bit of work, but it's worth it. To make it into a full meal, you could serve it with boiled eggs. In Andalusia in Spain, they often serve this with a few slices of Ibérico ham.

3 tbsp extra virgin olive oil

60g blanched almonds, roughly sliced

50g sourdough bread, roughly torn into chunks

250ml ice-cold water

400g ripe tomatoes

160g roasted red peppers from a jar, drained

1 garlic clove, peeled

1 tbsp sherry vinegar

Note

You will need to make this soup at least an hour before serving. However, it will keep in the fridge for up to 3 days when stored in an airtight container.

Heat the oil in a small frying pan over a medium heat, add the almonds and fry gently for about 4 minutes, until golden. Remove from the heat, tip the almonds and oil into a small bowl and set aside to cool.

Meanwhile, put the bread into a blender, pour over the cold water and leave to stand for 10 minutes.

Cut a small cross in the skin of each tomato, tip into a bowl and pour over enough boiling water to just cover. Leave to stand for 2 minutes, then drain and run under cold water for a minute; the skins should slip away easily. Squeeze the tomatoes over a bowl to collect the seeds (these can be discarded) then tip the flesh into the blender with the soaked bread.

Add the roasted peppers, garlic, sherry vinegar and a pinch of salt and pepper.

Spoon in most of the almonds and oil, saving a little for garnish, then blend on a high speed until completely smooth. Transfer to the fridge for at least an hour to chill, then pour into bowls and top with the reserved almonds and a drizzle of olive oil.

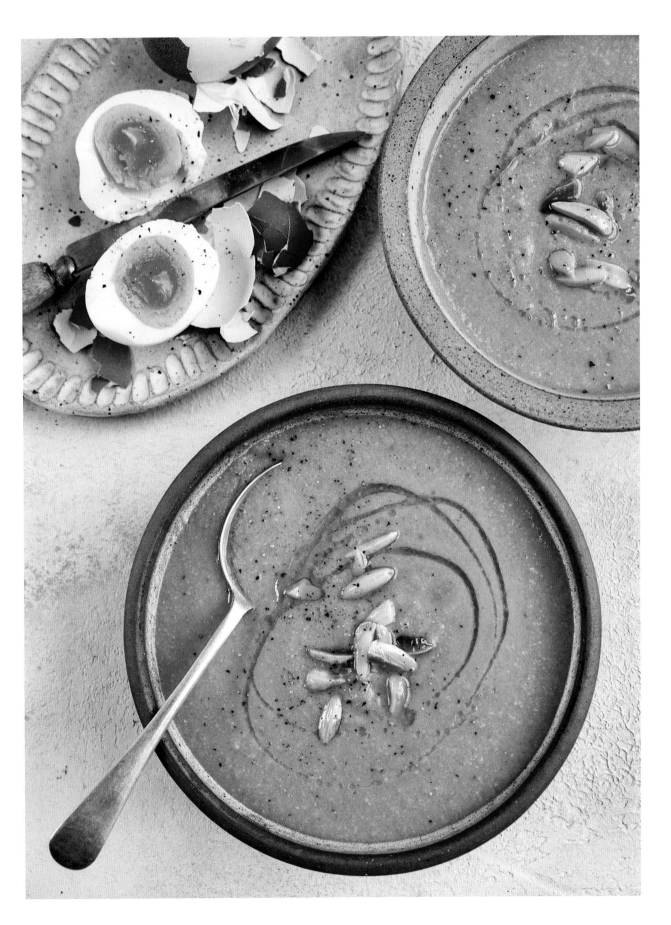

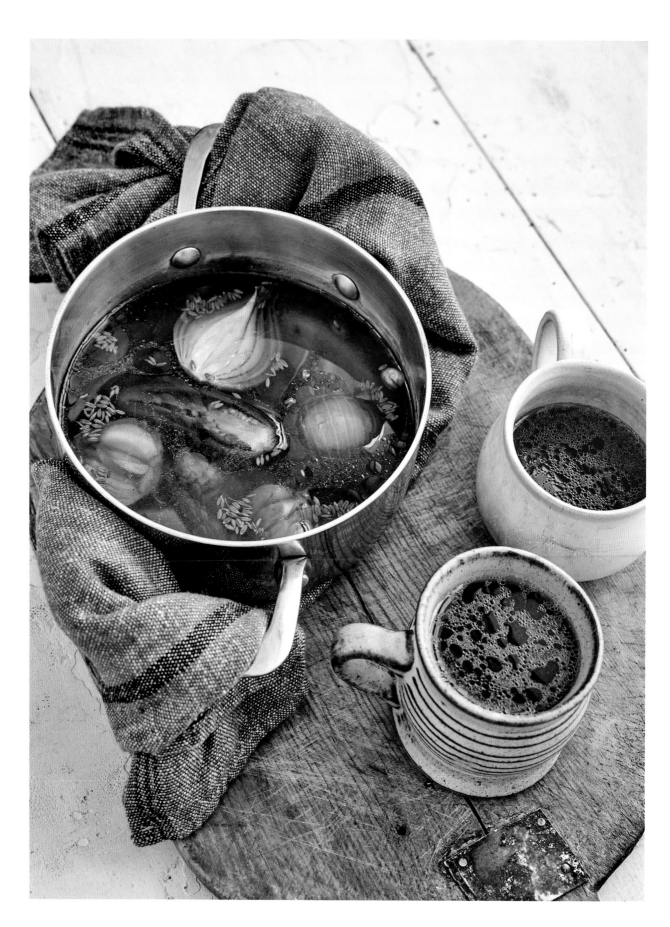

DR RUPY'S SIPPING BROTH

Makes 6 cups

Prep time: 5 minutes
Cook time: 35 minutes

This is a bit of a shared family recipe.
A gingery, spicy cup of broth that I always make whenever I feel slightly under the weather; it will certainly perk you up! It has a rich collection of plant chemicals known for their anti-microbial properties, such as garlic, onion, ginger and cinnamon. Personally, I swear by it for coughs and colds. Simple to put together and intensely warming.

2 red onions, peeled and halved

50g fresh ginger, roughly chopped

1 garlic bulb, halved crossways

1 green chilli, halved lengthways

1 tbsp extra virgin olive oil

5 green cardamom pods, bruised

1 tsp black peppercorns

4 cloves

1 tsp cumin seeds

1 cinnamon stick

Combine all the ingredients in a saucepan with 1.5 litres water and bring to a gentle simmer. Cook for 30 minutes, stirring occasionally. Remove the pan from the heat and strain the broth into a clean saucepan.

Season the broth to taste with salt. Ladle into mugs and sip hot, chilled or at room temperature throughout the day.

FENNEL & CHESTNUT SOUP

Serves 2

Prep time: 15 minutes
Cook time: 25 minutes

A simple collection of delicious flavours with one of my favourite and underrated ingredients, the humble chestnut. I use this all the time for its sweetness as well as its rich creaminess that gives a beautiful texture to any dish.

2 tbsp extra virgin olive oil

1 red onion (150g), roughly chopped

1 small fennel bulb (200g), roughly chopped

100g cooked chestnuts, crumbled

2 tsp nigella seeds

2 tsp fennel seeds

2 tsp dried oregano

1 litre boiling water

1 x 400g can cannellini beans, drained

1 vegetable stock cube

50g rocket, chopped

To serve

20g Parmesan or **vegetarian/ vegan Italian hard cheese**, finely grated

Small bunch of tarragon, chopped

Heat the oil in a large saucepan over a medium heat, add the onion, fennel and chestnuts and fry for 7 to 8 minutes until softened and beginning to caramelise.

Add the nigella and fennel seeds and the oregano, fry for a minute, then pour in the boiling water and add the beans and stock cube. Bring to the boil then reduce the heat and simmer for 15 minutes.

Remove the pan from the heat and use a stick blender to blend the soup until smooth. Stir through the rocket and leave it to gently wilt in the residual heat.

Ladle the soup into bowls and top with the Parmesan and chopped tarragon.

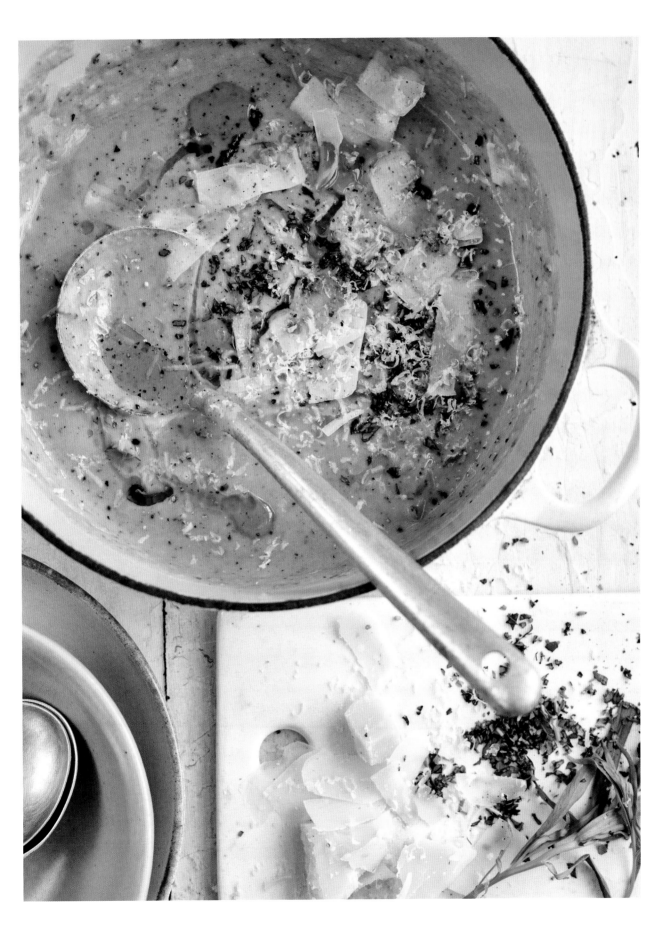

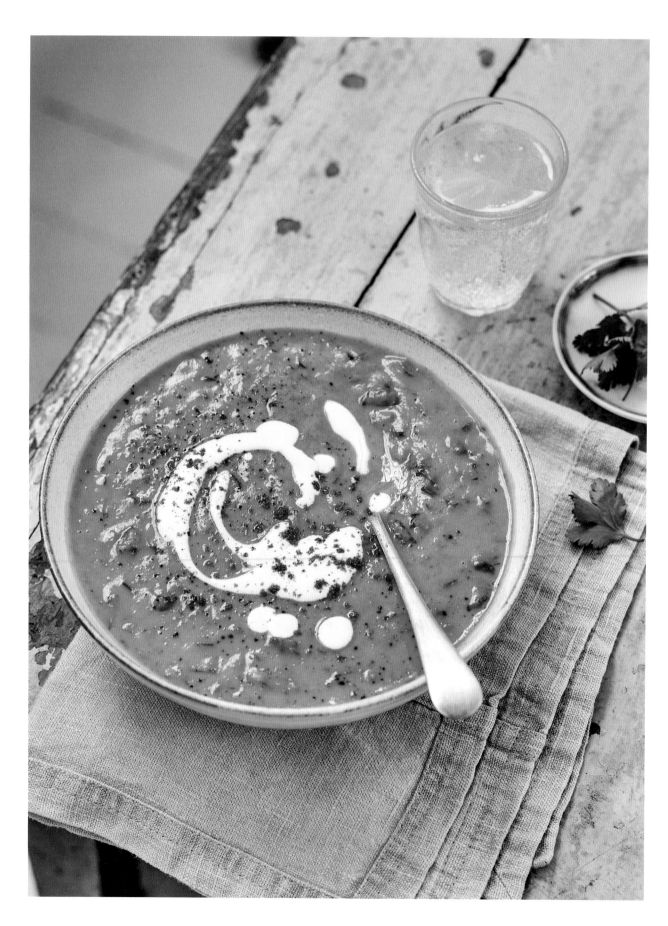

SWEET MASALA SOUP

Serves 2

Prep time: 10 minutes
Cook time: 35 minutes

This is a really comforting thick soup that is creamy with the lentils and sweet from the sautéed parsnips and sweet potato. The curry spices give a gentle undertone of warmth and the spinach and coriander mix at the end brings a freshness to the cooked vegetables. Almost four portions of vegetables per person, and plenty of flavour.

2 tbsp coconut oil

1 large red onion (150g), diced or sliced

20g fresh ginger, grated

2 tsp mild curry powder, plus extra to serve

½ tsp cardamom seeds, ground

1 large sweet potato (200g), scrubbed and left unpeeled, cut into 1cm cubes

2 small parsnips (200g), scrubbed and left unpeeled, cut into 1cm cubes

1 x 400g can green (or brown) lentils, drained and rinsed

1 tsp chilli flakes (or to taste)

750ml vegetable stock

5g coriander, chopped

50g spinach, finely chopped

2 tbsp unsweetened coconut yoghurt or **coconut cream**

Heat the coconut oil in a large saucepan over a medium heat and sauté the onion and ginger for 4 to 5 minutes.

Add the curry powder, cardamom, sweet potato and parsnips and cook for 10 minutes until softened and the spices have infused.

Add the lentils and chilli flakes, then cook for a further 2 minutes before adding the vegetable stock. Simmer for 10 to 15 minutes until the vegetables are soft.

Remove from the heat and blend with a stick blender; the soup should be thick.

Fold in the coriander and spinach and allow it to wilt in the heat of the pan.

To serve, ladle the soup into bowls, marble in some coconut yoghurt and dust with a pinch more curry powder.

CHILLI CORN CHOWDER

Serves 2

Prep time: 15 minutes
Cook time: 25 minutes

This is a really veg-heavy meal with deep, salty, umami flavours from the miso and stock that give a beautiful body to the corn. The beans add protein to this dish and the herbs work well with the sweet creaminess of the meal.

2 tbsp olive oil

200g celery, diced

150g green pepper, deseeded and diced

100g white onion, diced

1 tbsp miso paste

20g parsley, stalks and leaves separated and chopped

1 tsp dried tarragon

1 tsp dried oregano

1 tsp freshly ground black pepper

1 tsp cornflour

400ml vegetable stock

1 x 400g can butter beans, drained and rinsed

200g sweetcorn kernels (fresh or frozen and thawed)

1 tbsp chilli oil

Add the olive oil, celery, green pepper and onion with some seasoning to a large saucepan over a medium heat. Cook for 10 minutes until deeply coloured.

Add the miso paste, parsley stalks, dried herbs and ½ teaspoon of the black pepper, stirring for a further 1 minute to infuse the flavours into the vegetables.

Stir the cornflour into the vegetable mixture then pour in the stock with the beans and half the sweetcorn. Bring to a simmer for 10 minutes and then use a stick blender to blend the mixture together.

Add the remaining sweetcorn and black pepper and simmer for 3 minutes until the kernels are cooked but still with some bite.

Serve with a drizzle of chilli oil and the chopped parsley leaves scattered over.

Substitutions

Miso paste: 2 tbsp tamari

Green pepper: mushrooms (same weight as pepper)

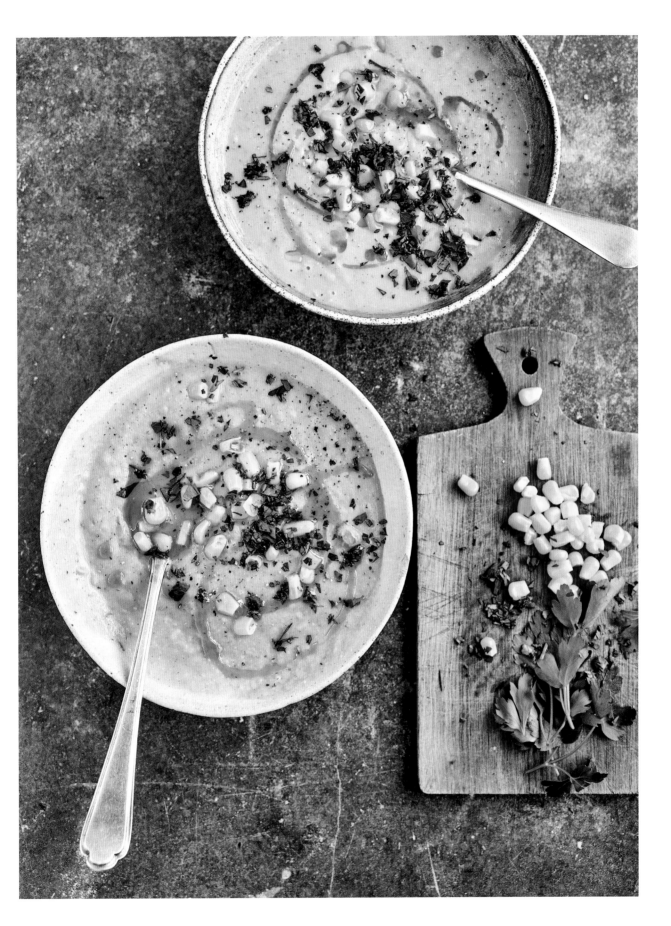

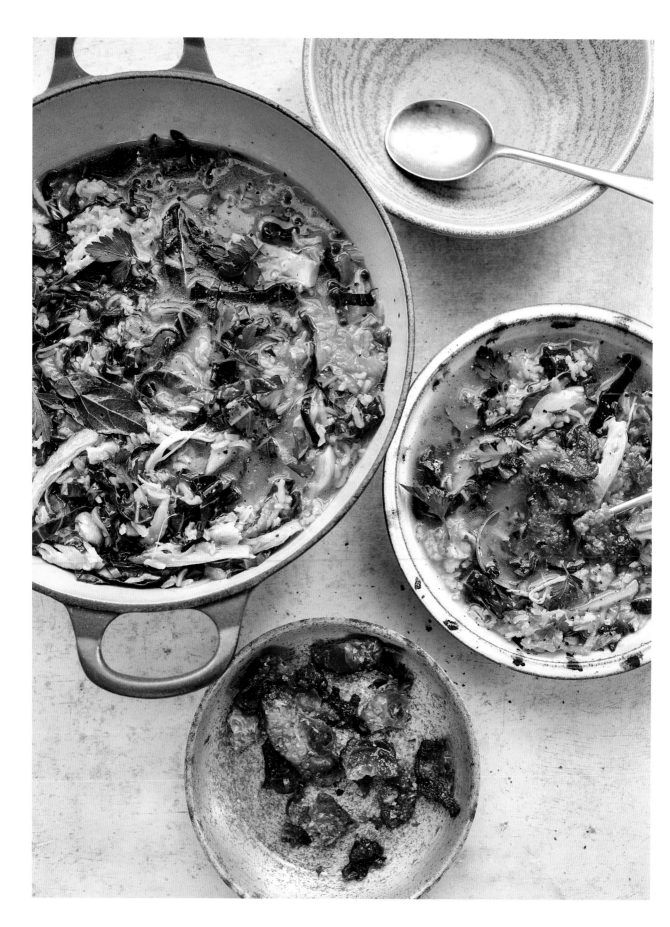

AYURVEDIC JEWISH PENICILLIN

Prep time: 15 minutes
Cook time: 45 minutes

This nourishing and spicy broth is my favourite meal to prepare for the family when they need a boost. It has a great collection of polyphenol-rich spices, anti-viral allium vegetables and plenty of warming flavours. I prefer to keep the spices like cloves and peppercorns whole, but feel free to remove them before serving.

2–3 bone-in chicken thighs (350g), skins removed and reserved (optional)

2 tbsp olive oil

1 large onion (180g), thinly sliced

3 celery sticks (175g), thinly sliced

6 garlic cloves, peeled and bashed

30g fresh ginger, sliced

2 bay leaves

4–5 thin slices of fresh turmeric or ½ tsp ground turmeric

2 tsp cumin seeds

2 tsp coriander seeds

1 tsp black mustard seeds

½ tsp black peppercorns

3 cloves

Small bunch of parsley, leaves and stalks chopped separately

100g brown basmati rice, thoroughly rinsed

1.2 litres chicken stock or **vegetable stock**

160g spring greens, finely shredded

Substitutions

Spring greens: spinach, pak choi or hispi cabbage

If serving with crispy chicken skin, preheat the oven to 180°C fan.

Spread the chicken skins flat on a baking tray, sprinkle with a little salt and roast in the oven for 20 minutes. Leave to stand (they will crisp up as they cool), then season lightly and break into shards.

Meanwhile, heat 1 tablespoon of the oil in a deep saucepan over a medium heat, add the chicken thighs and brown all over for 5 to 6 minutes. Remove from the pan and set aside.

Add the remaining oil to the pan and fry the onion and celery for 5 minutes until softened.

Add the garlic, ginger, bay leaves, turmeric and whole spices and fry for a further 1 minute.

Add the chopped parsley stalks and rice. Return the chicken to the pan then pour over the stock. Bring to a simmer, cover and simmer for 30 minutes. Add salt to taste (it may not need it if the stock was salty).

Remove the chicken from the pan and set aside to cool slightly. Pull the chicken meat from the bones, roughly chop, then put into individual bowls. Check for seasoning, add the shredded greens to the pan and simmer gently for a couple of minutes until wilted, then finish with the parsley leaves.

Ladle the soup into the bowls and top with shards of the crispy chicken skin, if you like.

CHIPOTLE CHICKEN & SWEETCORN SOUP

Serves 4

Prep time: 15 minutes
Cook time: 35 minutes

This thick, warming, smoky-flavoured soup is almost effortless. The chipotle paste does all the work, coating the chicken and vegetables in an aroma of spice that works beautifully with oregano and cinnamon. Unlike most chicken soups, this has bags of fibre and plenty of vegetables to deliver daily health benefits. Serve with toasted corn tortilla wraps or tortilla chips crushed over the top.

For the poached chicken

500ml boiling water

1 tbsp chipotle paste

2 chicken stock cubes

400g chicken breast fillet

For the soup

2 tbsp olive oil

4 celery sticks (240g), roughly chopped

250g shallots, roughly chopped

4 garlic cloves, grated

2 tsp dried oregano

1 tsp ground cumin

1 tsp ground cinnamon

1 tbsp chipotle paste

500ml boiling water

1 x 400g can pinto beans, drained and rinsed

400g sweetcorn (fresh, canned or frozen)

To serve

2–3 tbsp sliced jalapeños in brine from a jar

Small bunch of coriander, roughly torn

Pinch of smoked paprika

Pour the boiling water for the chicken into a saucepan, stir in the chipotle paste and stock cubes and bring to the boil. Add the chicken, bring back to a simmer, then cover and cook gently for 10 minutes. Strain the chicken, set aside to cool and reserve the poaching liquid.

While the chicken is poaching, add the oil to another large saucepan and set over a medium heat. Add the celery and shallots and cook for 6 to 7 minutes, until softened.

Add the garlic, oregano, cumin, cinnamon and chipotle paste, fry for 1 minute, then pour in the reserved poaching liquid and the boiling water.

Add the beans and sweetcorn, bring to a simmer and cook for 10 minutes. Meanwhile, shred the chicken using 2 forks.

Using a stick blender, blend the soup until smooth then stir in the shredded chicken. Ladle the soup into bowls and top with jalapeños, coriander and a pinch of smoked paprika.

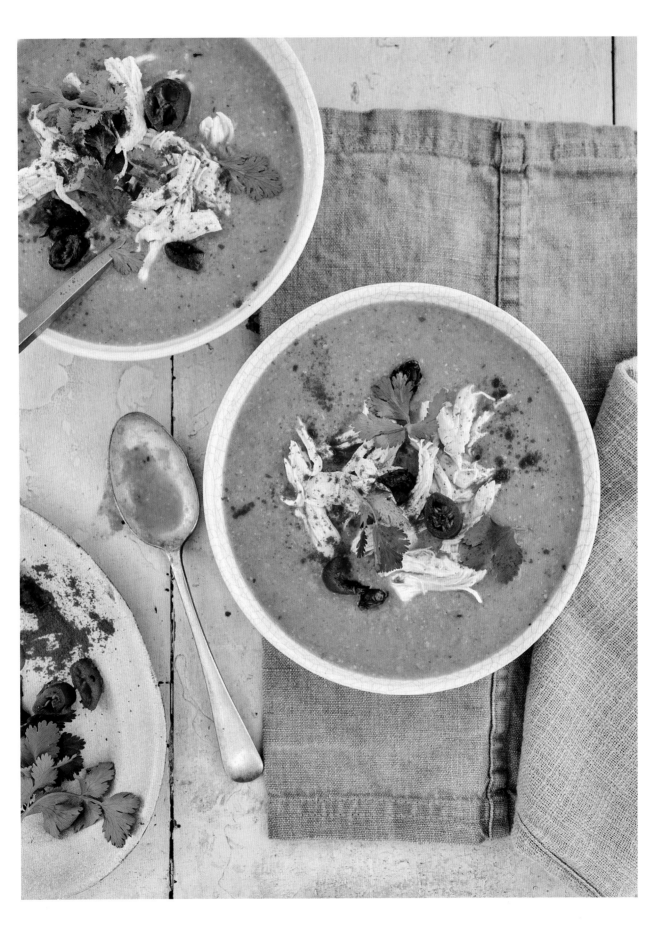

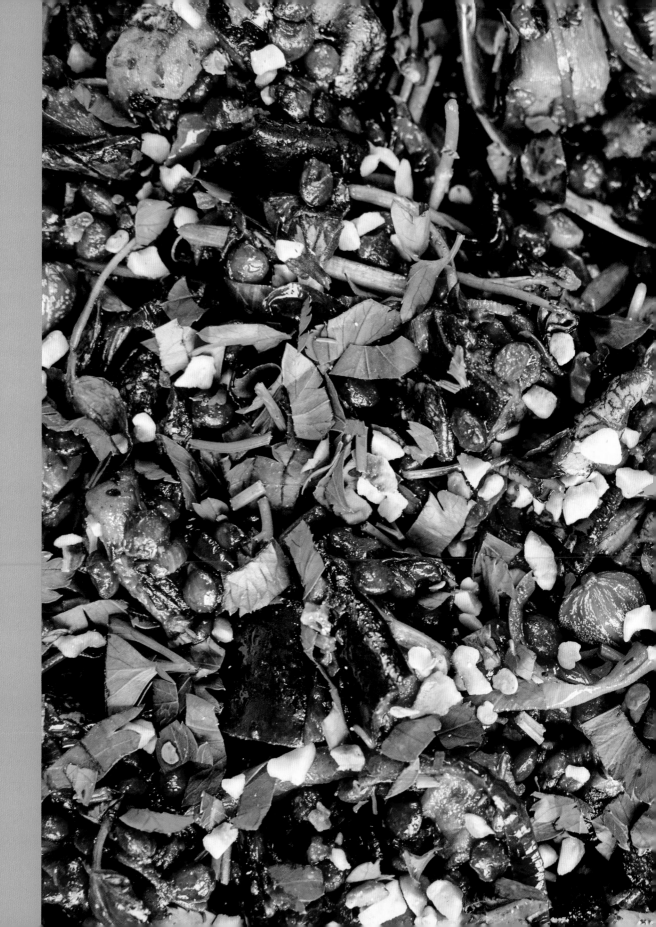

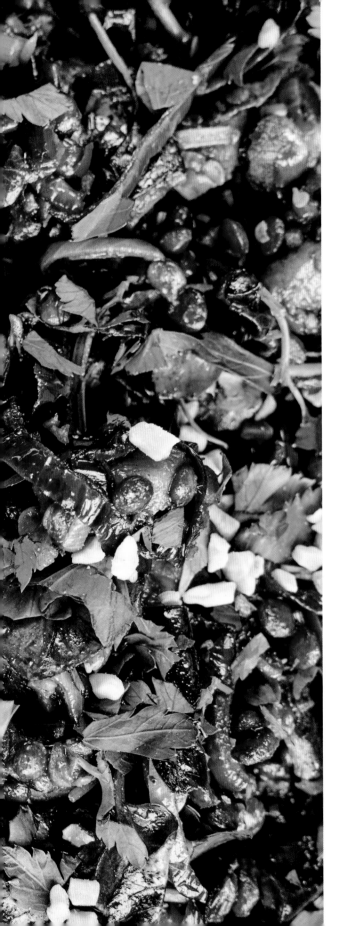

STIR FRIES & SAUTÉS

CELERY & BLACK BEAN STIR FRY

Serves 2

Prep time: 15 minutes
Cook time: 10 minutes

A satisfying stir fry with warm, spicy Sichuan pepper that coats the vibrant greens, rounded off beautifully with the perfume of Thai basil and the heat of chilli oil.

2 tbsp olive oil

3 celery sticks (180g), sliced on an angle, leaves reserved

1 tsp Sichuan peppercorns, crushed

3–4 dried red chillies, stems removed, roughly crumbled

4 garlic cloves, roughly chopped

200g cooked short-grain brown rice

200g tatsoi, roughly chopped

1 x 400g can black beans, drained

Small bunch of Thai basil, leaves roughly torn

For the sauce

2 tbsp tamari or **soy sauce**

1 tbsp rice vinegar

2 tsp chilli oil

1 tsp toasted sesame oil

Mix all the ingredients for the sauce together in a small bowl and set aside.

Heat the olive oil in a wok over a high heat, then add the celery, Sichuan pepper and dried chillies and fry for 2 minutes until lightly caramelised.

Add the garlic and rice, fry for 2 minutes then add the tatsoi. Fry for 1 or 2 minutes to wilt the leaves then add the black beans and fry for a further 1 minute.

Remove from the heat and stir through the sauce, celery leaves and Thai basil. Check the seasoning and serve.

Substitutions

Tatsoi: Swiss chard, kale, pak choi or choi sum

Short-grain brown rice: other wholegrain varieties

Sichuan peppercorns: plain black, green or red peppercorns

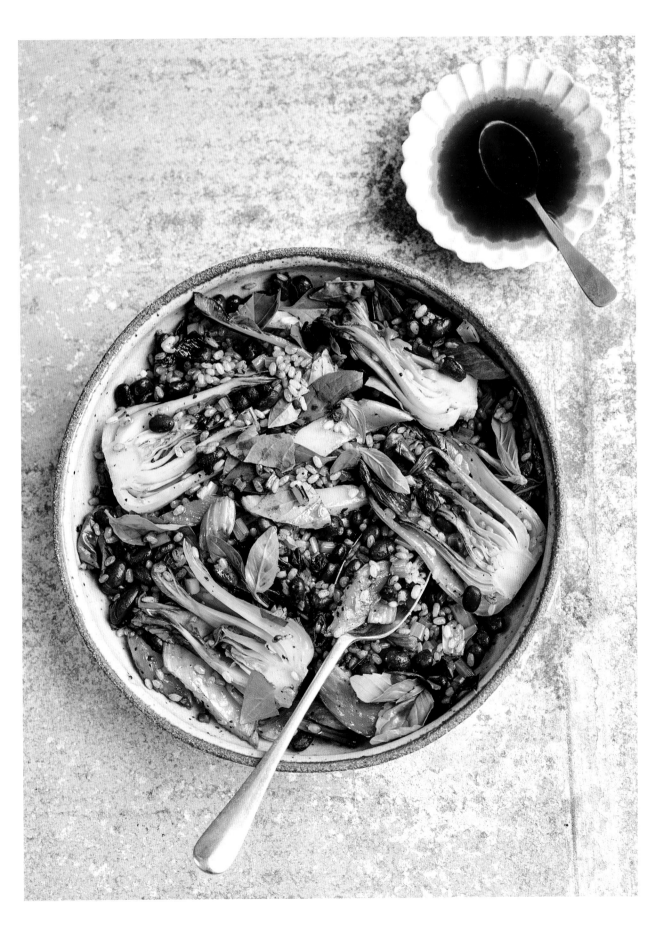

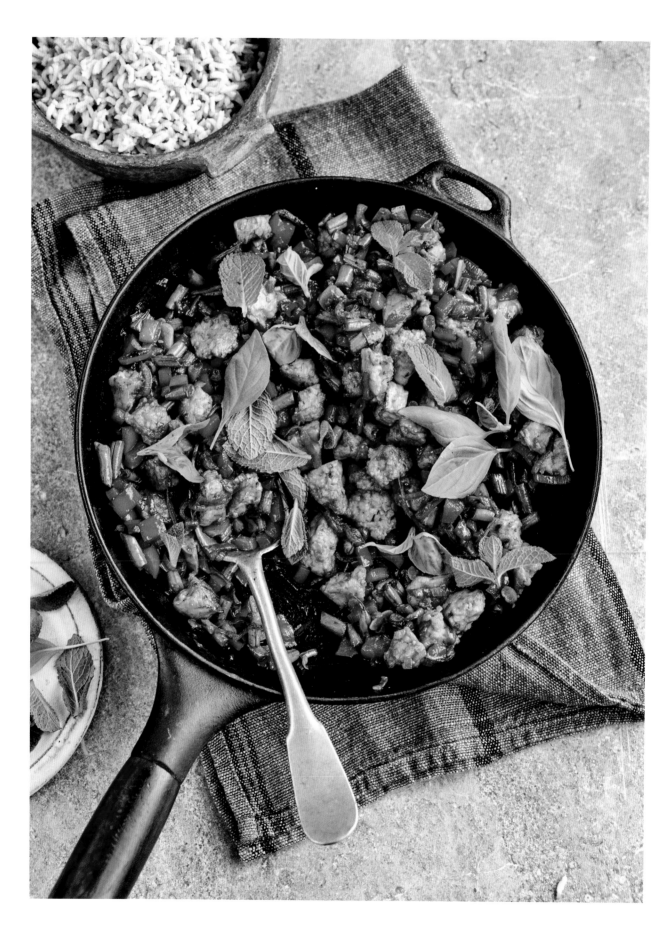

FRAGRANT & SWEET STIR FRY WITH HOLY BASIL

Serves 2 generously

Prep time: 15 minutes
Cook time: 20 minutes

My version of a pad kra pao that's typically made with pork mince. In this recipe tempeh is the star of the show; with its high fibre and protein content and ability to soak up flavour, I implore you to try it. It's delicious with these flavours and the aromatic sauce can be used in lots of variations. As a vegan and vegetarian alternative, use a mushroom sauce and omit the fish and oyster sauces..

2 tbsp sesame oil or **olive oil**

80g shallots, sliced

8 garlic cloves, sliced

1 red bird's-eye chilli, sliced

250g tempeh, crumbled into 2cm pieces

200g green beans, finely chopped

1 large red pepper (200g), deseeded and diced

10g Thai basil, leaves torn

10g mint, leaves torn

Juice of 1 lime

100g cooked short-grain brown rice

For the sauce

2 tbsp sesame oil

1 tbsp dark soy sauce

1 tbsp light soy sauce

2 tsp brown sugar

1 tsp cracked black pepper

1 tsp fish sauce (optional)

1 tsp oyster sauce (optional)

Mix all the ingredients for the sauce together in a small bowl.

Heat the oil in a large sauté pan over a medium heat, add the shallots and fry for 5 minutes until sweet and translucent. Add the garlic and chilli and cook for a further 3 minutes. Add the tempeh and cook for 5 minutes or until golden and browned all over.

Add the green beans and red pepper, reserving some red pepper to finish, and fry for a further 2 to 3 minutes, then add the sauce.

Cook for 5 minutes until the mixture is sticky and smelling delicious. Take off the heat.

Add the reserved red pepper, fold in the herbs, squeeze over the lime juice and serve over the rice.

Note

For a vegan version, omit the oyster and fish sauces or replace them with 2 tsp mushroom sauce.

GREENS IN A SPICY SESAME SAUCE

Serves 2

Prep time: 20 minutes
Cook time: 20 minutes

I love this sauce and so will you. I put it on everything and the combination of delicious umami flavours and the heat from garlic and chilli is perfect for jazzing up the tofu and fresh greens. The sauce makes double what you will need in this recipe, because it is great to keep for other greens, roasted vegetables or even a simple salad.

300g firm tofu, cut into 2cm cubes and patted dry

2 tsp cornflour

2 tbsp olive oil, plus a little extra

200g cavolo nero, stems removed, roughly chopped

200g fine green beans, halved

200g choi sum, stems chopped, leaves roughly torn

For the sauce (makes double)

100g toasted sesame seeds (or tahini)

4 tbsp olive oil

4 tbsp tamari or **dark soy sauce**

2 tbsp rice vinegar

4 tsp maple syrup

2 tsp toasted sesame oil

2 garlic cloves, peeled

2 tsp chilli flakes

Tip the tofu into a large bowl and dust with the cornflour.

Heat a large, lidded sauté pan over a medium heat and add the olive oil. Carefully add the tofu pieces and cook on all sides with a little salt for about 10 minutes or until golden brown and crispy. Tip onto a plate lined with kitchen paper and leave to crisp up.

Tip the cavolo nero and green beans into the same pan add some seasoning, toss in a little more oil and a splash of water, cover with a lid and cook for 8 minutes, adding the choi sum for the final 2 minutes of cooking.

Meanwhile, combine the ingredients for the sauce in a blender with 100ml water (or use a stick blender and a cup) and blend until smooth. The sauce should have the consistency of double cream; if it's a little too thick, add a splash of water.

Return the tofu to the pan with the vegetables, pour over half the sauce and quickly toss everything together. Transfer to a large serving bowl or platter and serve immediately.

The leftover sauce will keep for a week in the fridge, in an airtight container.

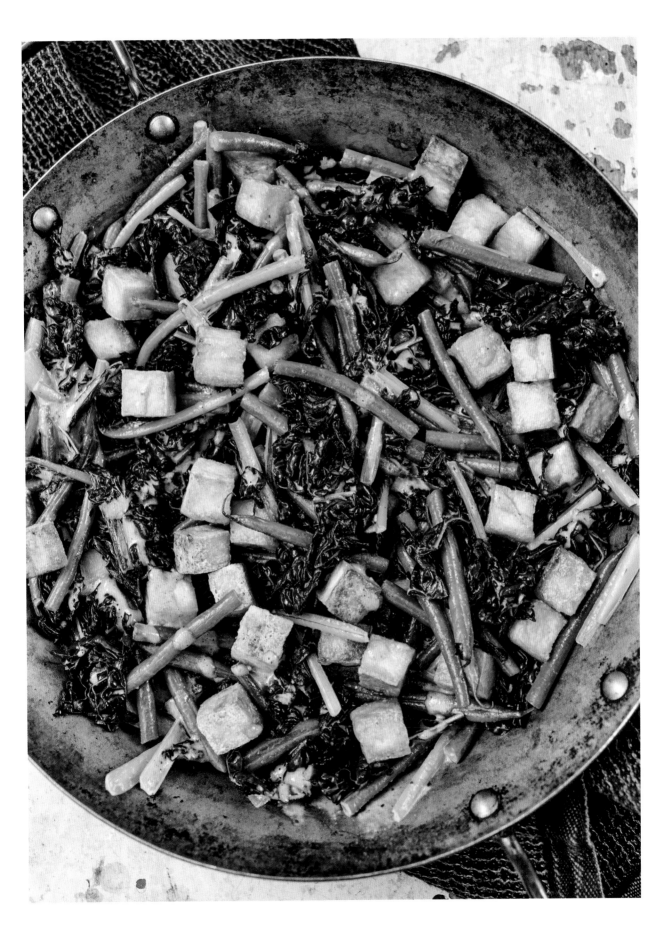

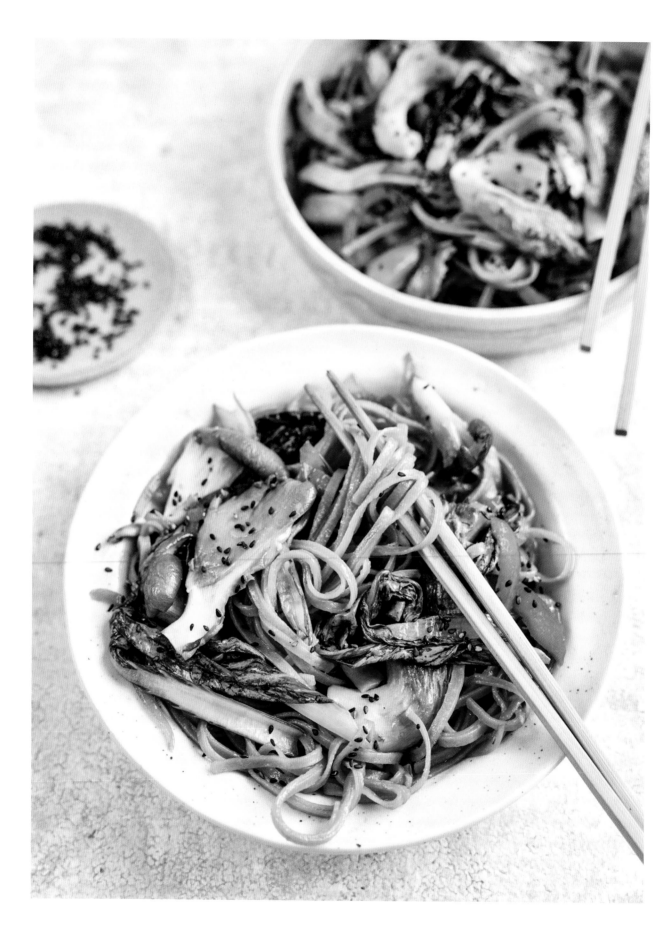

EASY NOODLES

Serves 2

Prep time: 15 minutes
Cook time: 20 minutes

A quick and simple dish that I love making during the week. You can easily swap the brown rice noodles for glass vermicelli noodles and if you're looking for more protein add tofu and some peanuts, but I love the simple mushroom, pepper and onion combination with the delicious and quick sauce.

150g brown rice noodles

160g oyster mushrooms, torn

2 tbsp extra virgin olive oil

1 onion (180g), sliced

1 green pepper (160g), deseeded and sliced

200g choi sum, shredded

20g black sesame seeds, to serve

50g kimchi, to serve

For the sauce

3 tbsp tamari or **soy sauce**

1 tbsp mirin

1 tbsp sesame seeds

1 tsp toasted sesame oil

1 tsp soft light brown sugar

2 garlic cloves, grated

½ tsp coarsely ground black pepper

Bring a large pan of water to the boil, add the noodles and cook for 5 to 6 minutes or according to the packet instructions. Drain and then rinse thoroughly under cold running water and set aside.

Combine all the ingredients for the sauce in a small bowl, whisk until the sugar has dissolved, then set aside.

Add the mushrooms to the wok and cook for 10 minutes or until golden and charred in places, then transfer to a plate lined with kitchen paper.

In the same wok, heat the oil over a high heat. Add the onion and pepper and stir-fry for 4 to 5 minutes or until softened and lightly charred. Add the choi sum and fry for 1 minute, then return the mushrooms to the wok with the noodles and sauce.

Quickly toss everything together over a high heat until combined. Serve with the sesame seeds scattered over and the kimchi on the side.

Substitutions

Brown rice noodles: vermicelli rice noodles or sweet potato noodles

Choi sum: pak choi, large leaf spinach or Swiss chard

SALT & PEPPER AUBERGINE

Serves 2

Prep time: 15 minutes
Cook time: 15 minutes

Tempeh is usually not on the top of everyone's ingredient list, but I personally love it for its ability to hold flavour, and of course for the health benefits of this protein and fibre-rich ingredient. Get some colour onto it and make it crispy, and it will soak up the delicious tart and chilli flavours in this dish really well.

2 tbsp olive oil

200g tempeh (gluten-free, if necessary), crumbled into jagged 1cm pieces

1 large aubergine (300g), cut into 1cm cubes

200g meaty mushrooms (king oyster or shiitake), finely chopped

2 garlic cloves, grated

30g fresh ginger, grated

1 small green chilli, thinly sliced

1 tsp coarsely ground black pepper

200g choi sum, stalks finely chopped, leaves shredded

2 tbsp kecap manis (or 2 tbsp tamari and 2 tsp brown sugar mixed together)

Small bunch of Thai basil, leaves only

20g unsalted roasted peanuts, roughly chopped

1 tsp toasted sesame oil

Heat the oil in a wok over a high heat. Add the tempeh and stir-fry for 4 to 5 minutes until golden and crisp.

Add the aubergine, mushrooms and a pinch of salt and stir-fry for 6 to 7 minutes, stirring regularly, until the vegetables are caramelised and soft.

Add the garlic, ginger, chilli and black pepper and stir-fry for 2 minutes until fragrant.

Stir through the choi sum and kecap manis and cook for a further 1 minute or so until the choi sum has wilted.

Remove from the heat and stir through the Thai basil and peanuts, and drizzle with a little sesame oil to serve.

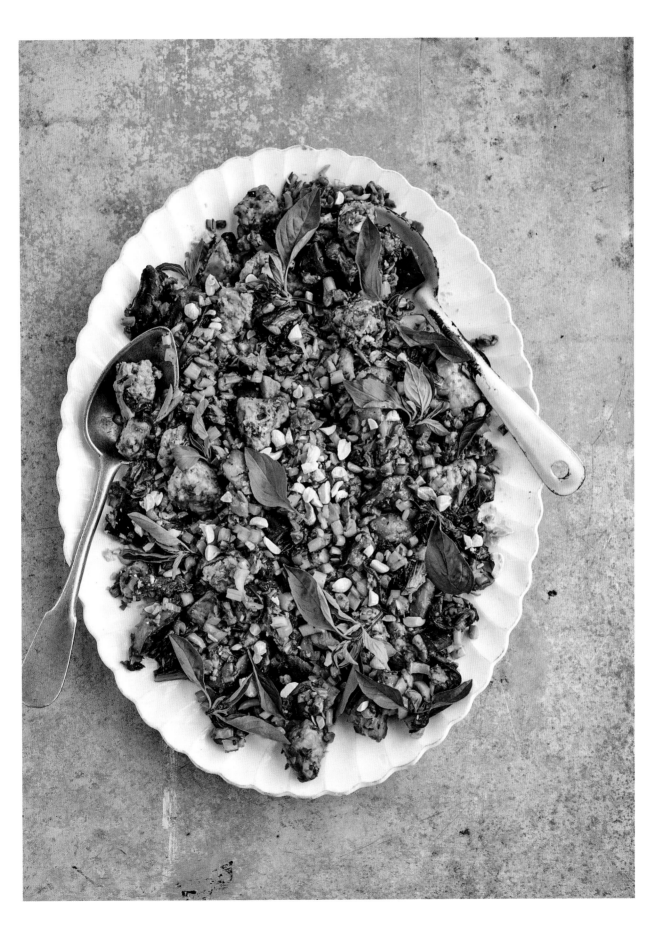

CRISPY SPICY MUSHROOMS WITH SWEET GREENS

Serves 2

Prep time: 20 minutes, plus 30 minutes standing
Cook time: 25 minutes

The rich spices pack heat, saltiness and a subtle sweetness into these mushrooms, which crisp up beautifully in the pan. The wilted greens, fresh parsley and quick pickle are welcome companions, rounding out the flavours, as well as bringing their individual health benefits. Ideally, I would cook all the ingredients in the same pan with the mushrooms, but to get that deep colour on them, they need their own space.

350g oyster mushrooms

1 tsp cumin seeds

1 tsp coriander seeds

1 tsp smoked paprika

½ tsp ground cinnamon

3 tbsp olive oil

2 tbsp tamari or **soy sauce**

1 tsp maple syrup

2 garlic cloves, grated

1 small white onion (100g), finely sliced

160g spring greens, roughly chopped

20g parsley, finely chopped

For the quick red cabbage pickle

100g red cabbage, finely shredded

1 tsp fennel seeds

50ml red wine vinegar

1 tsp brown sugar

1 tsp sea salt

50ml boiling water

To serve

Flatbreads

Tahini

Pickled jalapeños (from a jar)

For the quick red cabbage pickle, add all the ingredients except the boiling water to a bowl and massage them, using your fingers, for 1 minute. Pour over the boiling water and allow to stand for 30 minutes.

Tear the mushrooms into thin strips, then toss in a dry pan over a medium heat for about 8 minutes or until the liquid has largely evaporated and the mushrooms start to brown all over.

Pound the spices in a pestle with a mortar, then add to the mushrooms with 2 tablespoons of the olive oil. Sauté for 6 to 7 minutes until beginning to deeply colour and crisp up. Add the tamari or soy sauce, maple syrup and garlic, and cook for a further 3 to 4 minutes, until really dark and golden.

Remove the mushrooms from the pan and set aside. Add the onion and greens with the remaining oil to the same pan and sauté for 4 to 5 minutes until the greens have wilted. Throw in the parsley, stir and take off the heat.

Serve the mushrooms on warmed flatbreads with the greens and pickled cabbage, with a little tahini and pickled jalapeños.

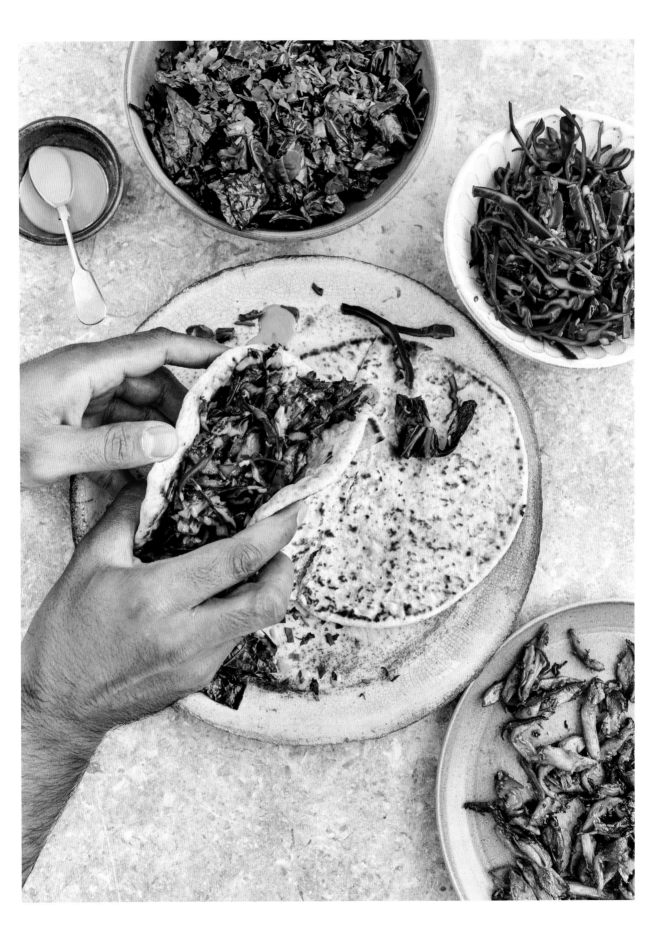

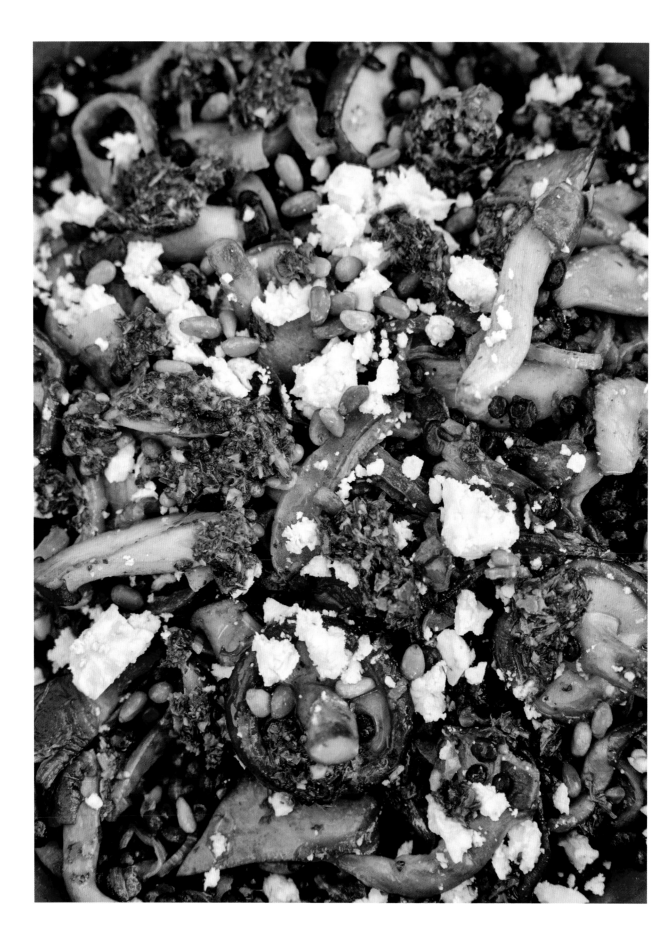

WILD MUSHROOMS WITH PUY LENTILS & SALSA VERDE

Serves 4

Prep time: 15 minutes
Cook time: 25 minutes

This sauté is packed with fresh flavour from the salsa verde and is super-simple to make. The green herb dressing adds a punch of colour and acidity to the sweet fennel and onions, and there's a good amount of protein and texture from the mushrooms. Serve with toasted sourdough, if you like.

4 tbsp olive oil

400g mixed wild mushrooms (oyster, Portobello or shiitake), sliced

1 large red onion (200g), peeled and thinly sliced

1 large fennel bulb (350g), thinly sliced

400g cooked Puy lentils

50g pine nuts, toasted

40g feta cheese (optional)

For the salsa verde

10g mint, leaves only

10g basil, leaves and stalks

10g parsley, leaves and stalks

1 tbsp capers, drained

1 garlic clove, grated

3 tbsp red wine vinegar

75ml olive oil

Heat half the oil in a large sauté pan or deep frying pan over a high heat, add the mushrooms and cook for 7 to 8 minutes or until soft and caramelised. (Depending on the size of your pan, you may have to do this in batches.) Transfer the mushrooms to a plate and set aside.

Add the remaining oil to the pan, reduce the heat slightly and add the onion and fennel. Cook for 10 to 12 minutes until soft and caramelised, then return the mushrooms to the pan. Stir in the lentils and season to taste.

For the salsa verde, put the herbs, capers, garlic and vinegar into a food processor and process, adding enough oil to create a loose sauce. Season with a pinch of salt.

Spoon the lentil and mushroom mixture onto a large platter, scatter over the toasted pine nuts and crumble over the feta, if using. Serve with the salsa verde.

Substitutions

Puy lentils: green, brown or beluga lentils

Pine nuts: sunflower seeds, pumpkin seeds, hazelnuts, walnuts

SPRING GREENS WITH ARTICHOKE

Serves 4

Prep time: 15 minutes
Cook time: 20 minutes

Light, crisp fresh vegetables with umami flavours and aniseed spicing, this is wonderful, easy and visually spectacular when you put it on the table. The tart artichoke flavours mellow gorgeously with the sweet leeks and garlic and the dish is formulated to have a good dose of prebiotic fibre per person. Good for your gut and great for your taste buds.

2 tbsp olive oil

300g leeks, roughly chopped

4 garlic cloves, diced

2 tsp nigella seeds

300g green beans, chopped

300g asparagus, chopped

200g peas (fresh or frozen)

150g artichoke marinated in vinegar (from a jar), chopped

1 tbsp white miso paste

50ml white wine

1 tsp cracked black pepper

100g spinach, finely chopped

Small bunch each of mint and parsley (5g), finely chopped

Heat the oil in a lidded pan over a medium heat and sauté the leeks and garlic for 8 minutes, seasoning well.

Add the nigella seeds, green beans and asparagus, stirring through the cooked leeks for about 1 minute, then pop the lid on for 3 to 4 minutes to cook them through.

Add the peas, replace the lid and cook for a further 1 minute, then add the chopped artichoke, miso paste, wine and black pepper. Cook, with the lid off, for 3 minutes.

Fold in the chopped spinach and herbs, take off the heat and allow them to wilt in the residual heat of the pan before serving.

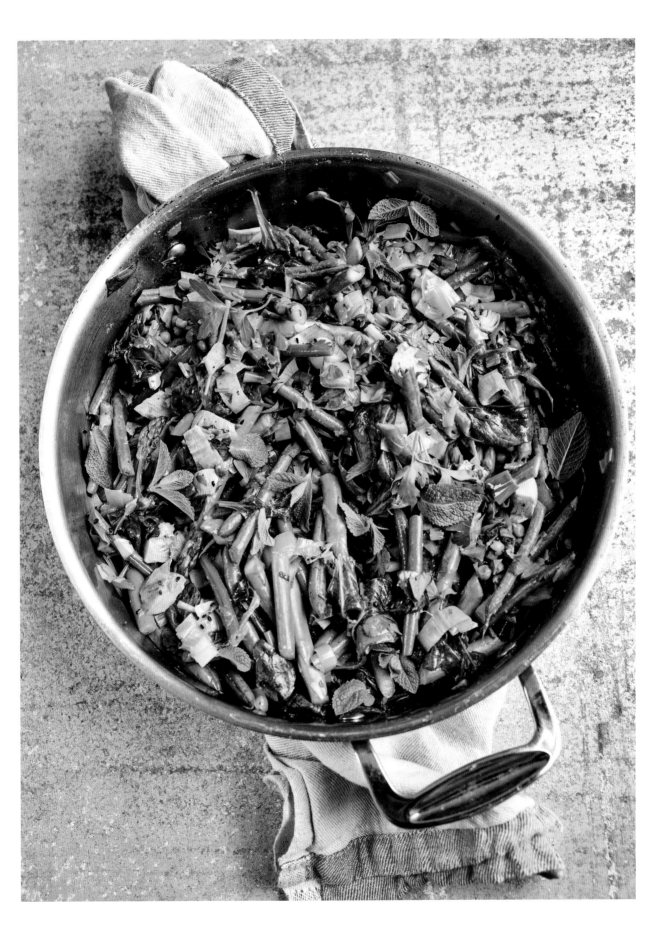

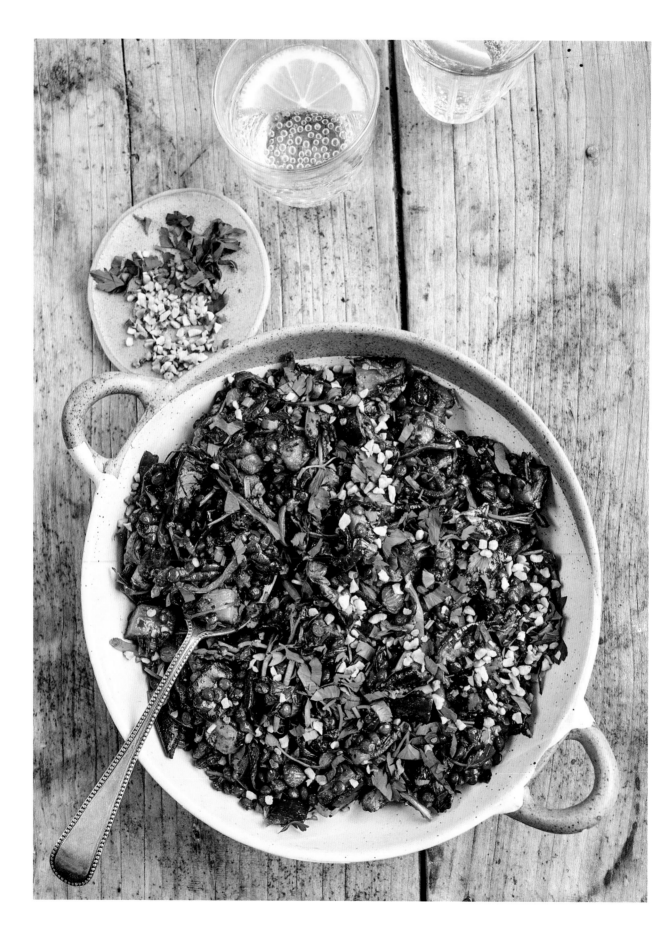

AUBERGINE SAUTÉ WITH BALSAMIC VINEGAR & PINE NUTS

Serves 2

Prep time: 15 minutes
Cook time: 20 minutes

This is sort of like a caponata without the tomatoes because I want a bit more texture to the meal rather than a sauce, although you could very easily add tomatoes to this dish. The salty, sweet and tart marriage of capers, onion and balsamic vinegar transports you to the southern Mediterranean. This works really well on toasted sourdough or even with a little pasta.

1 large aubergine (300g), cut into 1cm cubes

3 tbsp olive oil

4 garlic cloves, diced

150g red onion, thinly sliced

20g capers or **pitted black olives**

2 tsp dried oregano

25g parsley, stalks and leaves separated and chopped

½–1 tsp chilli flakes

1 tbsp balsamic vinegar

200g cooked Umbrian lentils (or beluga, Puy or brown lentils)

100g watercress, chopped

30g pine nuts or **crushed hazelnuts,** toasted

Fry the aubergine in a dry pan for 7 to 8 minutes over a medium heat until it slightly chars in places. Then add the oil, garlic and onion and sauté for 8 to 10 minutes until softened.

Add the capers, oregano, parsley stalks, chilli flakes, balsamic vinegar and lentils and stir through the ingredients for 1 minute.

Add the watercress and cook for 1 minute to wilt gently, then finish with the toasted pine nuts or crushed hazelnuts and the parsley leaves.

YAKISOBA WITH EDAMAME & MUSHROOMS

Serves 2

Prep time: 15 minutes
Cook time: 10 minutes

Rather than reaching for a takeout app, I think about whether I have the ingredients for this super-satisfying and quick stir fry… and I usually do! The rich, tangy sauce is a perfect combination for bright vegetables, protein-rich edamame and mushrooms. This recipe is hard and fast, so grab a wok or large sauté pan and turn up the heat.

150g ramen noodles or **buckwheat soba noodles**

1 tbsp sesame oil

2 tbsp olive oil

1 carrot (100g), peeled and cut into thin matchsticks

1 red pepper (100g), deseeded and thinly sliced

200g shiitake mushrooms, thinly sliced

2 garlic cloves, peeled and roughly sliced

160g shelled edamame beans

For the sauce

2 tbsp Worcestershire sauce or **mushroom sauce**

1 tbsp oyster sauce (optional)

1 tbsp mirin

1 tbsp sriracha

2 tsp dark soy sauce or **tamari**

1 tsp light brown soft sugar

To serve

4 spring onions (50g), finely sliced on an angle

2 tbsp pickled ginger

1 tbsp aonori (flaked nori seaweed, optional)

Whisk all the ingredients for the sauce together in a small bowl and set aside.

Bring a pan of water to the boil, add the noodles and cook for 1 minute less than directed on the packet instructions. Drain and rinse under cold water, then tip into a bowl and toss with the sesame oil.

Heat the olive oil in a wok over a high heat. Add the carrot and pepper and stir-fry for 2 minutes, then add the mushrooms and garlic. Stir-fry for 3 minutes until the mushrooms have softened and taken on some colour.

Stir the edamame beans and noodles through the stir-fried vegetables. Fry for a further 1 to 2 minutes, then pour over the sauce and let everything bubble up for 30 to 60 seconds.

Divide the noodles between two bowls, top with the spring onions, pickled ginger and seaweed flakes, and serve.

Substitutions

Mushrooms: oyster, king oyster or chestnut mushrooms

Seaweed flakes: seaweed snacks simply torn into pieces

Note

For a simpler (and vegan) version of the sauce, use just mirin and soy or tamari, and double the quantities

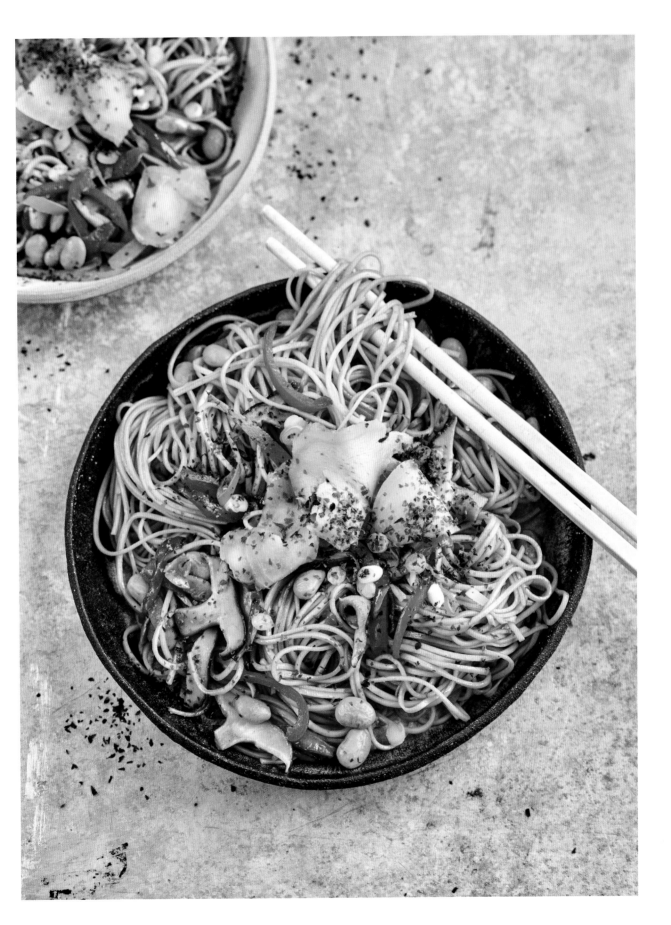

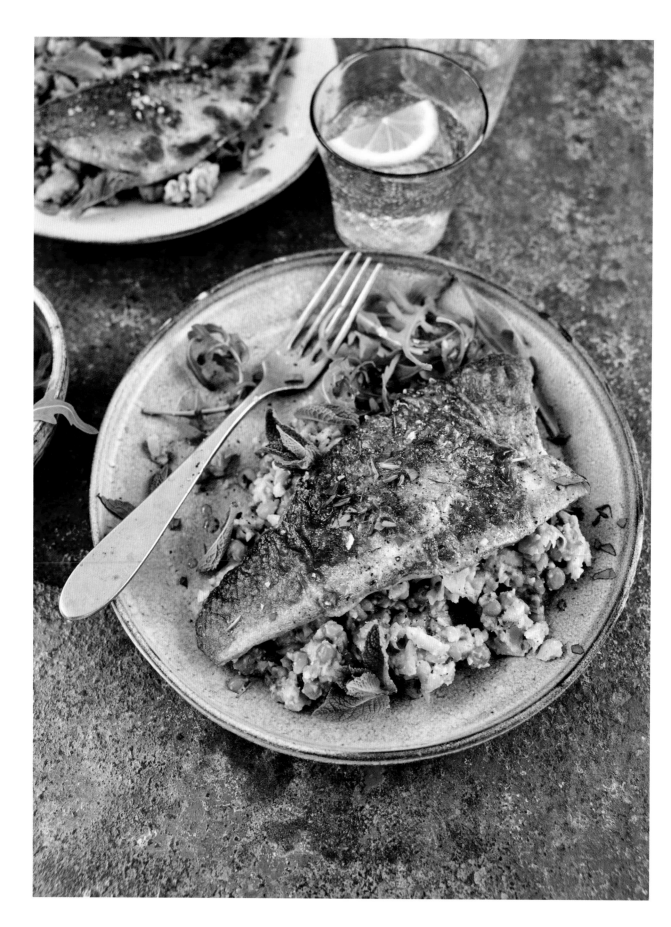

CRISPY SEABASS WITH MASHED PEAS

Serves 2

Prep time: 15 minutes
Cook time: 15 minutes

This is a quick and simple favourite of mine. When you want something that is easy, adaptable and foolproof, this is ideal. It has plenty of greens and ample fibre, as well as the gentle sweet heat from the pepper, fennel and cayenne combination.

2 seabass fillets (about 300g)

2 tbsp rice flour

½ tsp cayenne pepper

1 tsp fennel seeds, roughly ground

1 tsp freshly ground black pepper

3 tbsp olive oil

100g rocket, roughly chopped

Juice of 1 lemon

For the peas

200g peas (fresh or frozen)

1 x 400g can butter beans, drained and rinsed

2 tsp miso paste

1 garlic clove, grated

10g tarragon leaves, chopped

10g mint leaves, chopped

Black pepper

Pat the fish fillets dry with kitchen paper. Mix the flour with the spices and a pinch of salt on a plate and coat the fish in the flour mixture, dusting off any excess.

Place a frying pan over a medium heat, add the olive oil and gently place the fish skin-side down in the pan, lightly pressing the flesh to prevent the fillets from curling at the edges.

Cook for 5 minutes until the skin is crispy, then flip and cook for a further 1 minute on the other side. Leaving the pan on the heat, remove the fish from the pan and place on kitchen paper to soak up any excess oil.

Lower the heat. To the same pan, add the peas, butter beans, miso paste, garlic, some black pepper and a splash of hot water. Stir together, cover with a lid and cook for 4 to 5 minutes, then stir in the fresh herbs.

Using the back of a fork or a potato masher, roughly crush the peas and beans in the pan.

Plate the crushed peas and beans and top with the rocket leaves, tarragon and mint. Place the fish fillets on top and squeeze over some fresh lemon.

Substitutions

Seabass: any similar fish fillet, such as sea bream, tilapia or sole

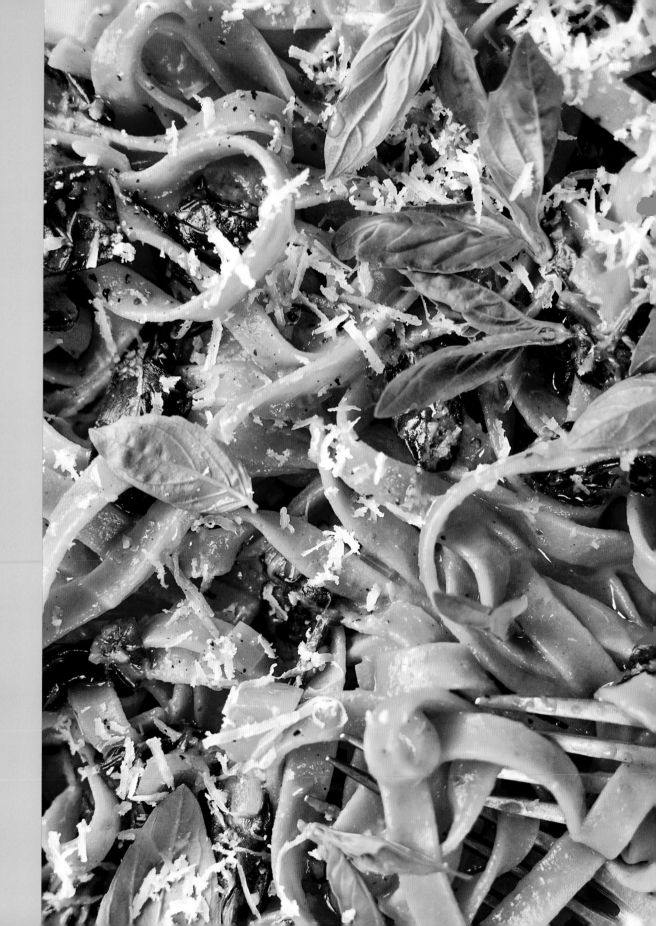

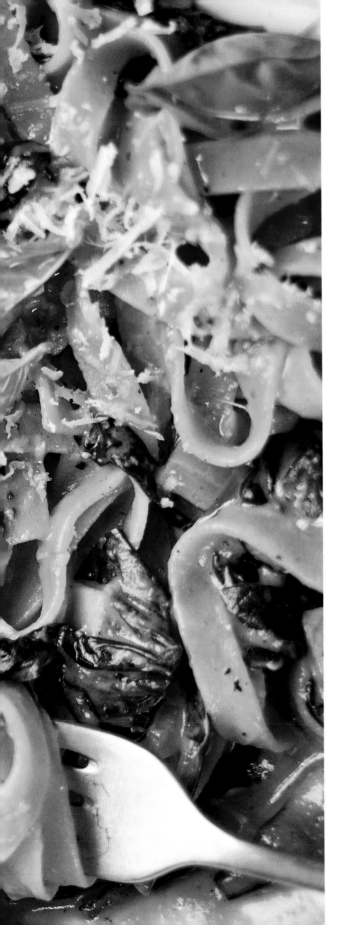

RICE & PASTA

INAUTHENTIC SINGAPOREAN CHICKEN RICE

Serves 4 generously

Prep time: 20 minutes
Cook time: 1 hour 40 minutes

A take on Hainanese chicken, with wonderful aromatic flavours, delicious spices and plenty of colourful greens to serve with a gorgeously flavoured rice. Cooking a chicken in this way is super economical and low waste, as well as bringing out the best from the produce.

1 x 1.5kg chicken

50g fresh ginger, sliced

6 garlic cloves, unpeeled, bashed

4 tbsp tamari or soy sauce

2 tbsp coriander seeds

2 tsp black peppercorns

3 star anise

6 cloves

300g short-grain brown rice, rinsed well

To serve

400g choi sum or pak choi

300g ripe tomatoes, diced

1 cucumber, thinly sliced

4 spring onions, shredded

Small bunch of coriander, torn

4 tbsp Cheat's Quick Chilli Oil or Chinese chiu chow chilli oil (shop-bought)

Put the chicken into a large stockpot and pour over enough cold water to completely cover. Add the ginger, garlic, tamari or soy sauce and spices, then bring to a gentle simmer. Cover and cook for 40 minutes, skimming the surface occasionally to remove any impurities. Remove from the heat and leave to stand with the lid on for 10 minutes, then transfer the chicken to a baking tray, cover loosely with foil and set aside to rest.

Strain the poaching broth into a jug, skim off any fat, then pour 600ml back into the pan (any leftover broth can be chilled or frozen). Add the rice, bring to the boil, then reduce to a gentle simmer, cover with a lid and cook for 30 minutes. Remove from the heat and leave to stand with the lid on for a further 10 minutes.

When the rice is nearly ready, steam the choi sum or pak choi in a separate pan for 2 to 3 minutes until wilted.

Take the chicken breast off the bone and cut into thick slices. Pull the thigh and leg meat away from the bone. Season the rice with a little extra tamari or soy sauce, if needed. Serve the chicken with the rice, choi sum, tomatoes and cucumber, drizzled with the chilli oil. Garnish with the spring onions and coriander.

3 tbsp light olive oil

1 tsp toasted sesame oil

2 tsp tamari or light soy sauce

½ tsp brown sugar

1 garlic clove, grated

½ tsp chilli flakes

CHEAT'S QUICK CHILLI OIL

Combine all the ingredients in a small saucepan and warm gently until the garlic starts to fizz. Remove the pan from the heat, stir for 1 minute then leave to cool.

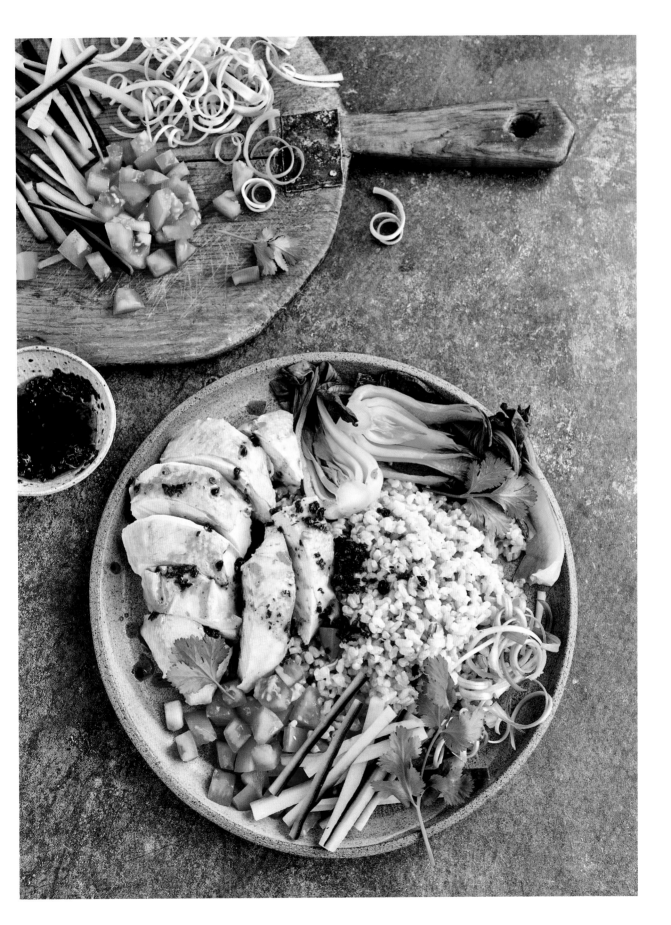

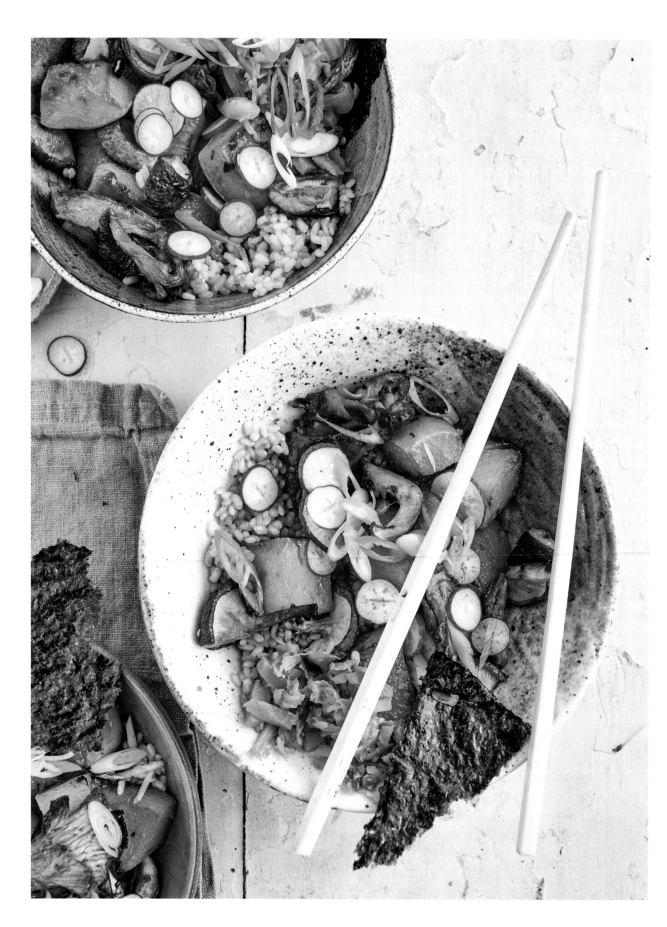

MISO-ROASTED MUSHROOM DONBURI

Serves 2 or 3

Prep time: 15 minutes
Cook time: 30 minutes

The combination of sweet butternut squash in a rich umami paste, with the sharp kimchi and meaty mushrooms, works beautifully. The marinade is so easy to make in the pan and can be used on a variety of vegetables. This meal packs in over three portions of vegetables per serving, making this a delicious way to hit your plant density goals.

1 tbsp **white miso paste**

2 tbsp **tamari** or **light soy sauce**

1 tbsp **maple** or **agave syrup**

1 tbsp **sesame oil** or **light olive oil**

½–1 tsp **chilli flakes**

300g mixed mushrooms, roughly torn (I use shiitake and oyster)

300g butternut squash, skin on and deseeded, cut into 2cm cubes

250g short-grain brown rice, well rinsed

370ml boiling water

1 tbsp **mirin**

1 tbsp **rice vinegar**

To serve

5g nori seaweed snacks, torn

80g kimchi

80g radishes, thinly sliced or cut into thin matchsticks

80g spring onions, thinly sliced on an angle

Preheat the oven to 200°C fan.

Add the miso, tamari or soy, maple or agave syrup, oil and chilli flakes to a large bowl and whisk together. Add the mushrooms and squash and toss until thoroughly coated.

Add the squash to a roasting tray and bake for 15 minutes. Remove the tray from the oven, turn the squash pieces, move to one half of the tray and add the marinated mushrooms. Bake for another 15 minutes until cooked and lightly caramelised.

Meanwhile, tip the rice into a dry saucepan over a medium heat. Toast the grains lightly for a minute until they are dry. Pour in the boiling water and simmer with the lid on for 20 minutes. Remove from the heat, leave to stand, covered, for 10 minutes, then stir in the mirin and vinegar. Season the rice with a little extra tamari or soy sauce, if needed.

To serve, spoon the rice into individual, deep bowls, then arrange the seaweed, kimchi, radishes, spring onions and miso-roasted mushroom and squash on top.

Notes

Roast the seeds from the squash at the same time with a little oil, salt and pepper for a snack.

To increase the protein content, add precooked edamame beans to the topping, or tempeh.

WILD MUSHROOM RICE WITH FENNEL & COURGETTE

Serves 2

Prep time: 20 minutes
Cook time: 50 minutes

A delicious mix of wholegrain rice, earthy mushrooms and a balance of punchy herbs and spices make this a satisfying and comforting meal. The tamari and red wine vinegar balances the dish well and the parsley adds a freshness at the end.

30g dried wild mushrooms, such as porcini or ceps (75g rehydrated weight)

500ml boiling water

150g mixture of brown basmati and wild rice, rinsed well, soaked for 10 minutes then drained

2 tbsp extra virgin olive oil

1 small fennel bulb (200g), thinly sliced

1 courgette (190g), halved lengthways and cut into 5mm slices

4 celery sticks (220g), thinly sliced

2 garlic cloves, grated

60g pumpkin seeds

1 tsp fennel seeds

1 tsp sweet paprika

1 tsp dried oregano

2 tbsp tamari

1 tbsp red wine vinegar

15g parsley, roughly chopped

Substitutions

Brown basmati and wild rice mixture: brown rice, short-grain brown rice or venus rice

Tip the mushrooms into a bowl, pour over the boiling water, cover and leave to stand for 20 minutes.

Using a slotted spoon, transfer the mushrooms from the soaking liquid into a clean bowl. Next, using a ladle, carefully spoon most of the soaking liquid into a measuring jug; leave the last bit of soaking liquid in the bowl as it usually contains grit from the mushrooms.

Add the rice to a dry saucepan over a medium heat and toast the grains for 2 to 3 minutes to bring out its nutty flavour. Pour 300ml of the mushroom soaking liquid into the pan, bring to the boil and cover with a lid. Reduce the heat to low and simmer gently for 20 minutes. Remove the pan from the heat and leave to stand for 10 minutes with the lid on.

Meanwhile, heat the oil in a deep frying pan over a medium heat. Add the fennel, courgette and celery, season lightly and fry for 7 to 8 minutes until golden. Increase the heat slightly, add the mushrooms, garlic, pumpkin seeds, fennel seeds, paprika and oregano and fry for 2 to 3 minutes. Remove the pan from the heat.

To serve, fold the cooked rice, tamari, vinegar and parsley into the mushroom and vegetable mixture.

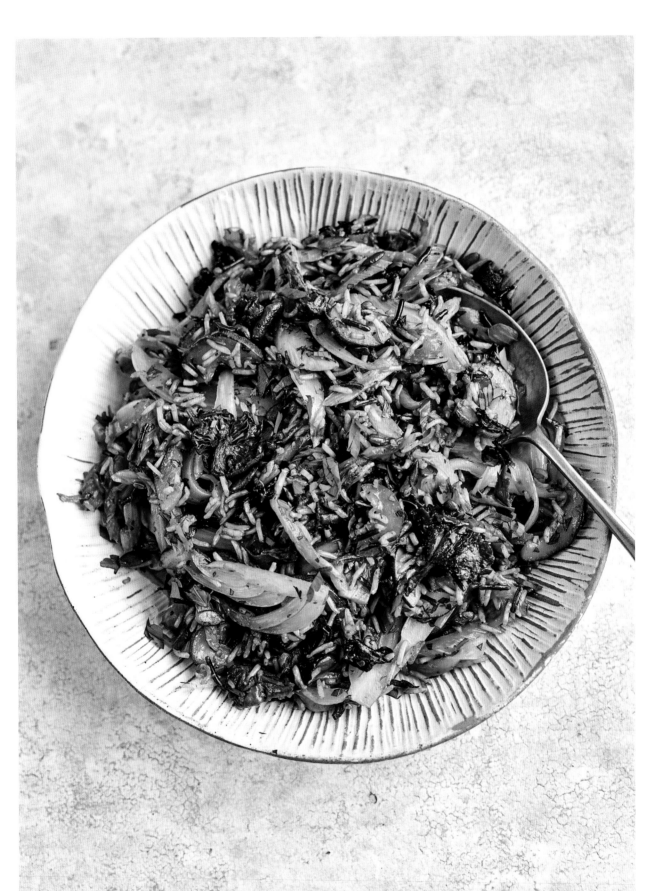

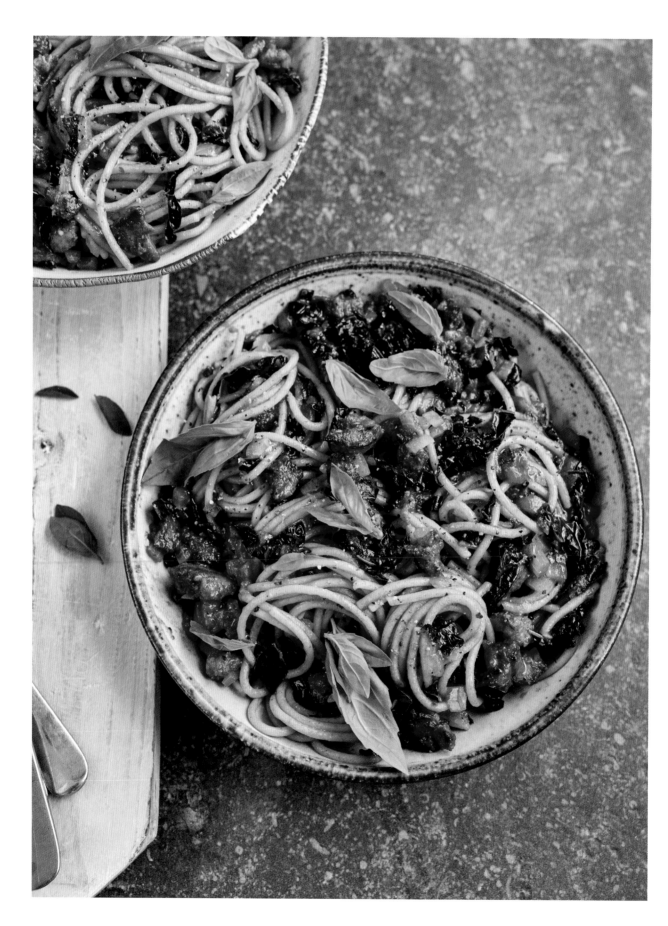

DR RUPY'S SPAGHETTI

Serves 2

Prep time: 15 minutes
Cook time: 40 minutes

I can't call this a bolognese, so I'm just calling it mine. You may be tempted to skip this recipe on account of one ingredient, but tofu prepared using this method is absolutely divine. It has a rich, deep flavour and a texture that resembles crispy ground beef. I now cook tofu this way all the time. Give it a go.

120g wholewheat spaghetti

160g cavolo nero, stems removed and leaves finely sliced

10g basil leaves, chopped, plus extra whole leaves to serve

For the spicy ground tofu

300g extra-firm tofu (see Note)

1 tsp ground cumin

1½ tsp smoked paprika

½ tsp ground cinnamon

1 tsp dried oregano

Pinch of salt

1 tsp ground black pepper

3 tbsp dark soy sauce

1 tbsp date molasses or maple syrup

2 tbsp olive oil

For the sauce

2 tbsp olive oil

4 garlic cloves, diced

1 white onion (160g), finely diced

20g tomato purée

1 x 400g can chopped tomatoes

1 tbsp balsamic vinegar

Note
To improve the texure of tofu, wrap in kitchen paper, place a cast-iron pan (or other heavy weight) on top and leave for 30 minutes.

Preheat the oven to 200°C fan.

First dry out the tofu by crumbling it into a roasting tin and mashing it with a fork into small pieces. Place in the oven for 5 minutes to dry out any excess moisture but remove it just before the tofu starts to stick to the tin.

Add the remaining spicy ground tofu ingredients to the tin and mix thoroughly. Spread out into an even layer and bake in the oven for 20 to 25 minutes, stirring occasionally to prevent sticking. The tofu should be dry and charred in places, resembling cooked ground beef in both look and texture.

Meanwhile, to make the sauce, heat the oil in a saucepan over a medium heat. Add the garlic and onion with some seasoning and fry gently for 5 minutes until soft. Add the tomato purée, chopped tomatoes and vinegar, and cook with the lid on for 20 minutes until sweet and thick.

Bring a large pan of salted water to the boil, add the spaghetti and cook according to the packet instructions. Drain the pasta, reserving some of the cooking water.

Loosen the sauce with the reserved pasta cooking water. Add the cavolo nero, cover with a lid and cook for 5 to 6 minutes until wilted.

To finish, stir most of the spicy ground tofu and the chopped basil through the tomato sauce, then add the drained spaghetti and toss everything together. Serve in bowls, garnished with the remaining crispy tofu and a few extra basil leaves.

VEGGIE PAPPARDELLE

Serves 4

Prep time: 20 minutes
Cook time: 60 minutes

For me, this is a take on a ragù, but as my extended Italian family always remind me, it can't be a ragù without all the meat, so I have to refrain from calling it that. Jackfruit works really well as a plant-based option to add texture to this dish. The final result with all the herbs is unctuous and satisfying.

2 x 400g cans jackfruit, drained and rinsed

2 tbsp olive oil, plus extra to drizzle

2 small white onions (200g), finely diced

2 small carrots (200g), finely diced

4 garlic cloves, finely diced

1 tsp chilli flakes

½ tsp grated nutmeg

1 sprig of rosemary, leaves chopped

2 tsp dried thyme

2 tsp dried oregano

1 bay leaf

100ml red wine

2 x 400g cans plum tomatoes (or chopped tomatoes)

2 tbsp tomato purée

1 vegetable stock cube

1 tbsp miso paste (optional)

400g wholewheat pappardelle

250g cavolo nero, stems removed and leaves finely chopped

20g Parmesan, pecorino or vegetarian/vegan Italian hard cheese, grated (optional)

Substitutions

Cavolo nero: spring greens, kale or hispi cabbage

Jackfruit: borlotti beans

Preheat the oven to 220°C fan.

Scatter the jackfruit pieces over a large baking tray, drizzle with some of the olive oil and season well. Bake in the oven for 30 minutes or until browned and it easily pulls apart like pieces of stringy meat.

Meanwhile, heat the 2 tablespoons of oil in a large saucepan over a medium heat. Add the onions, carrots and garlic and sauté for 8 minutes until softened.

When the jackfruit is baked, pull the pieces apart and add to the pan along with all the spices, herbs and some seasoning. Stir for 1 minute. Pour in the wine, then add the tomatoes and tomato purée. Crumble in the stock cube, add the miso, if using, and stir to combine, then bring to a gentle simmer. Cover with a lid and cook for 20 minutes to allow the flavours to mingle and intensify.

While the sauce is cooking, bring a large pan of salted water to the boil, add the pappardelle and cook according to the packet instructions.

Fold the cavolo nero into the sauce for the last 5 minutes of the cooking time, so that it wilts in the sauce.

Drain the pappardelle and serve with the veggie sauce and topped with grated cheese, if you like.

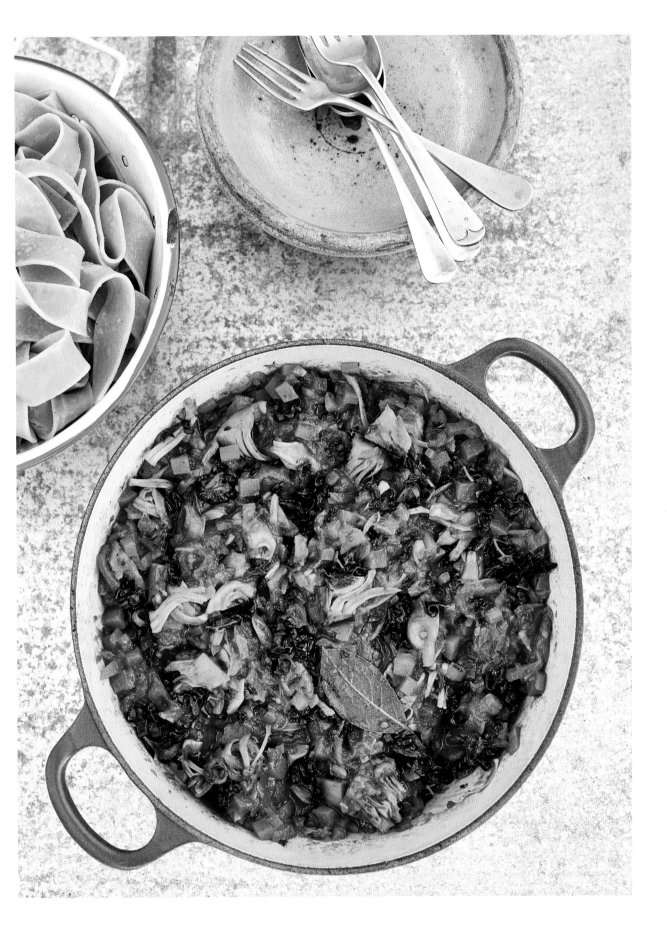

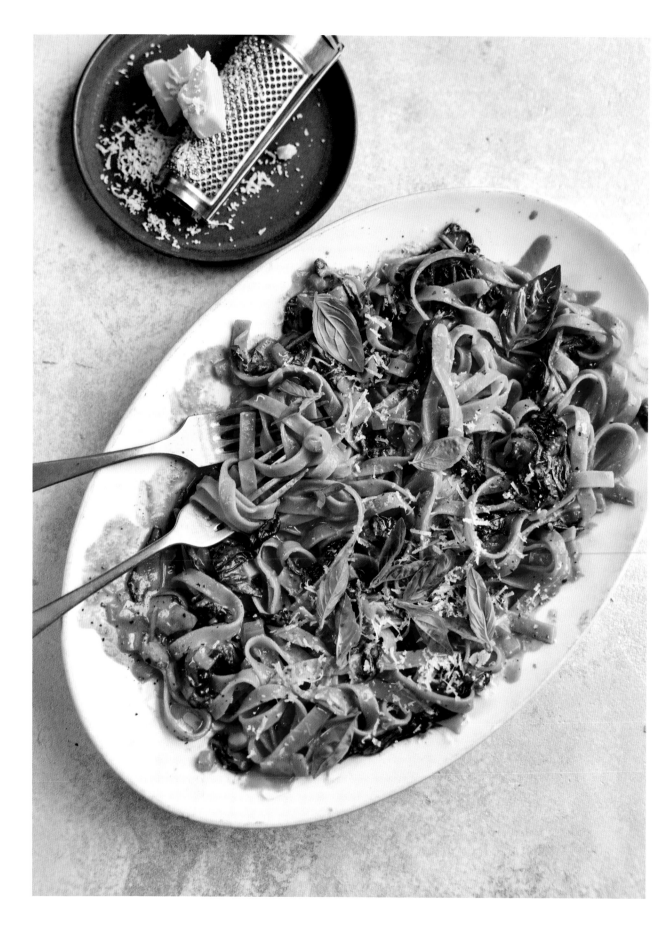

ROAST PEPPER PASTA

Serves 2

Prep time: 10 minutes
Cook time: 15 minutes

You might feel sceptical about adding silken tofu to your pasta, but trust me, it really works in this sauce and it tastes delicious. Plus you get the added benefits of a high-protein ingredient with novel plant chemicals shown to reduce inflammation, as well as a creamy and delicious texture to your pasta. If you need this dish to be vegan, then omit the Parmesan grated over the top – it will still be absolutely delicious.

150g dried tagliatelle (preferably wholewheat)

2 tbsp extra virgin olive oil, plus extra to serve

1 onion (160g), chopped

2 garlic cloves, grated

200g large leaf spinach

For the sauce

4 large roasted red peppers (240g) from a jar, drained and roughly chopped

150g silken tofu

2 tbsp tamari or **soy sauce**

Pinch of black pepper

1 tsp chilli flakes

To serve

Small bunch of basil, leaves torn

20g Parmesan, pecorino or **vegetarian/vegan Italian hard cheese**, grated (optional)

Bring a large pan of salted water to the boil, add the pasta and cook according to the packet instructions.

Meanwhile, to make the sauce, tip all the ingredients into a blender and blitz until smooth.

Heat the oil in a sauté pan or deep frying pan over a medium heat. Add the onion, garlic and a pinch of salt and fry gently for 6 to 7 minutes until soft. Increase the heat, add the spinach and cook for 2 minutes until wilted.

Drain the pasta, reserving a little of the cooking water. Pour the blended sauce into the pan with the onions and spinach and cook for 1 minute, stirring continuously. Add the cooked pasta to the pan and toss to combine until all the pasta is coated in the sauce. If the sauce is a little thick, loosen with a splash of the reserved pasta cooking water.

To serve, spoon the pasta into bowls, drizzle over a little olive oil and scatter over the basil leaves and grated cheese, if using.

BYZANTINE SPICED PRAWN SPAGHETTI

Serves 2 with leftovers

Prep time: 20 minutes
Cook time: 25 minutes

This colourful spaghetti dish has an adventurous use of spices that work beautifully with fresh seafood to give a light, aromatic flavour to the pasta. The allium vegetables take on the polyphenol-rich spices well and the pistachios give a lovely extra texture to the dish. I've packed this with prebiotic-rich ingredients like onion and celery, which slows the digestion of carbohydrates and reduces sugar spiking from typical heavy pasta dishes.

3 tbsp extra virgin olive oil

3 celery sticks (160g), diced

1 small fennel bulb (200g), diced

1 onion (180g), diced

120g wholewheat spaghetti

Small bunch of parsley, stalks and leaves separated and chopped

4 garlic cloves, grated

1 cardamom pod, seeds crushed

1 tsp coriander seeds, crushed

1 tsp ground ginger

½–1 tsp chilli flakes

½ tsp ground cinnamon

Pinch of ground nutmeg

60g shelled pistachios, finely chopped

150ml dry white wine

250g raw jumbo prawns, shelled and deveined

Juice of 1 lemon

Heat 2 tablespoons of the oil in a shallow, flameproof casserole over a medium-high heat. Add the celery, fennel and onion and cook gently for 10 minutes, stirring regularly, until softened and caramelised.

Meanwhile, bring a large pan of salted water to the boil, add the spaghetti and cook according to the packet instructions.

Add the parsley stalks and garlic to the casserole, then stir in the spices with half of the pistachios. Sauté for a further 2 to 3 minutes until fragrant, then pour in the wine and let everything bubble up for a couple of minutes.

Add the prawns to the pan and cook for about 4 minutes or until pink all over. Drain the pasta, reserving some of the cooking water. Add the spaghetti to the pan along with a ladleful of the pasta cooking water and a pinch each of salt and pepper.

Add the chopped parsley leaves, toss everything together, then serve topped with the remaining pistachios, lemon juice and olive oil.

Substitutions

Prawns: shrimp or crab

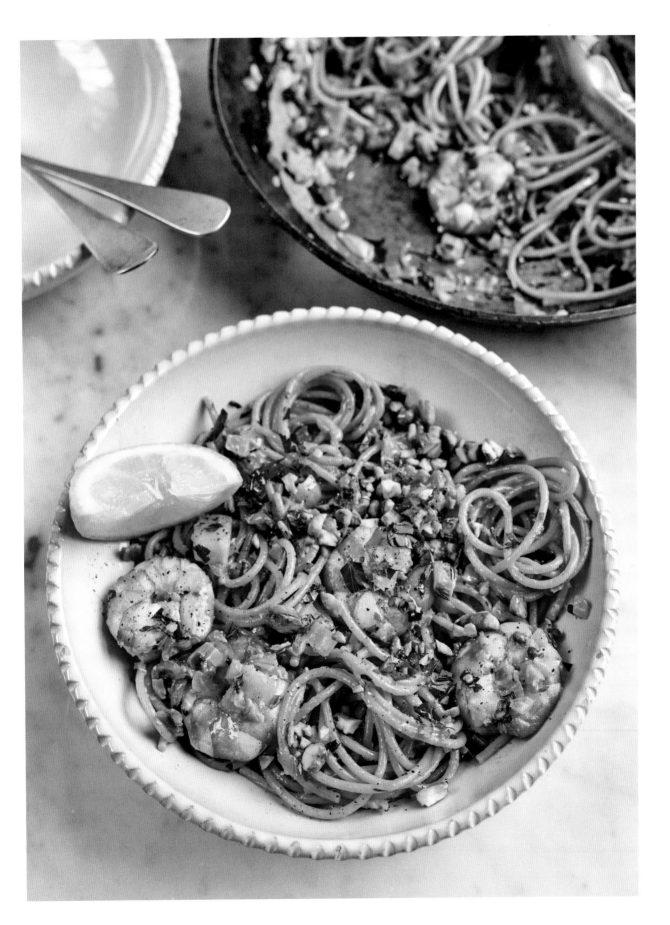

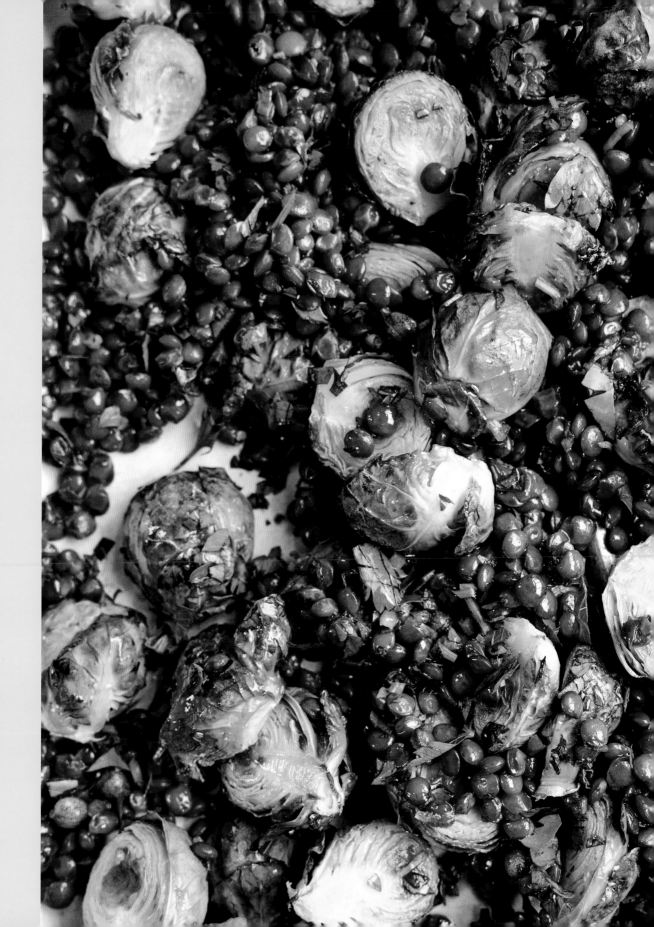

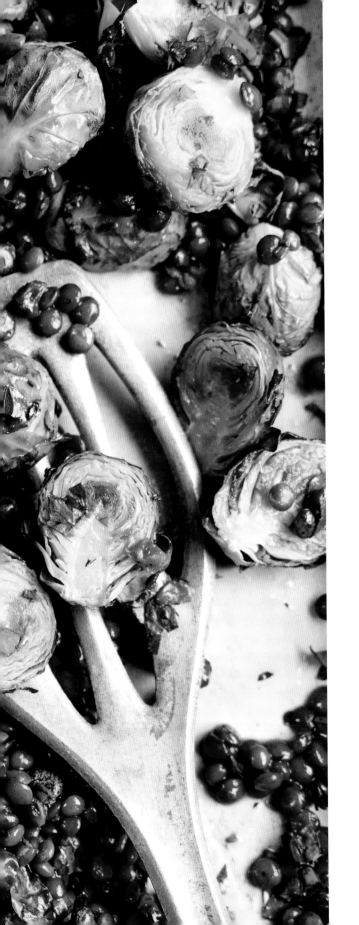

LIGHT MEALS, SIDES & SALADS

BLACK-EYED BEANS WITH ROCKET

Serves 4 as a side salad

Prep time: 5 minutes
Cook time: 20 minutes

The surprising combination of spices delivers a wonderful smoky flavour, with a background of sweetness that pairs beautifully with the fibre and protein-rich beans. For such few ingredients, there is a wealth of punchy flavour in the finished dish!

2 tbsp tamari or **dark soy sauce**

2–3 tbsp olive oil

2 tsp nigella seeds

2 tsp cumin seeds

1 x 400g can black-eye beans, drained and rinsed

100g rocket leaves, roughly chopped

100g pomegranate seeds

Substitutions

Black-eyed Beans: borlotti beans, white beans

Pomegranate: orange segments

Preheat the oven to 180°C fan.

Whisk the tamari or soy sauce, olive oil and spices together in a large bowl, add the beans and some salt and pepper to taste, and toss to coat.

Tip into a large roasting tin, shake out into an even layer then bake for 20 minutes, stirring halfway through the cooking time, until almost all of the liquid has gone.

Leave the beans to cool for a few minutes then tip into a large bowl, add the rocket and pomegranate seeds and toss together. Check the seasoning, spoon into bowls and serve.

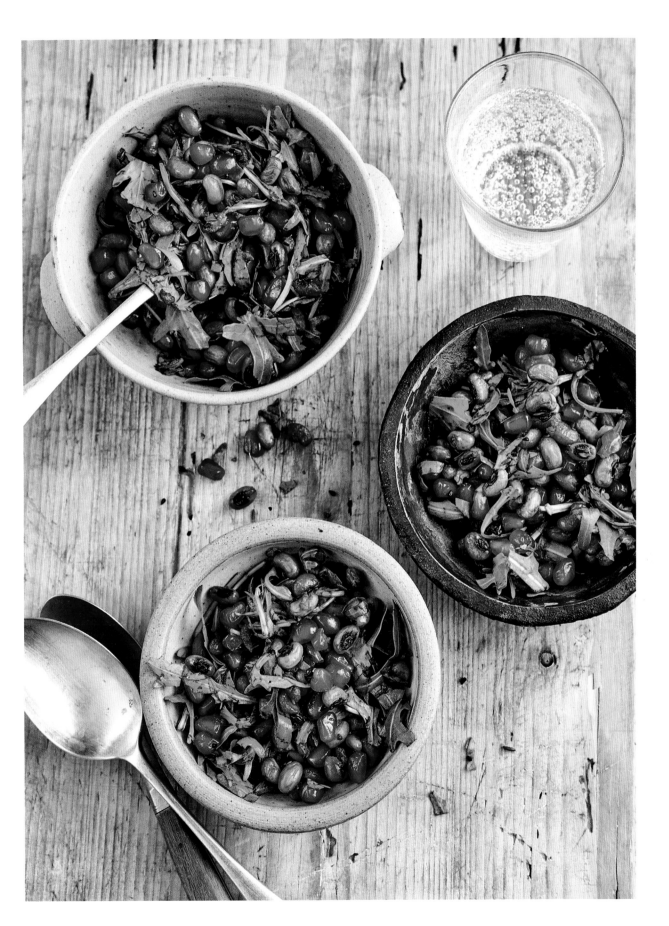

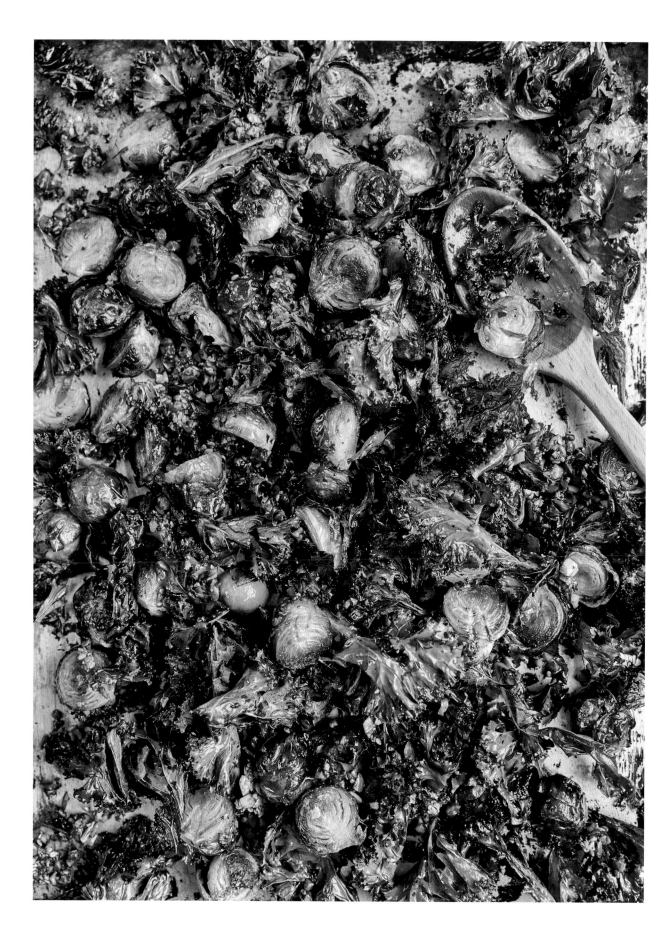

CHARRED BRUSSELS WITH SPICY PEANUT SAUCE

Serves 2

Prep time: 15 minutes
Cook time: 30 minutes

The combination of flavours in this spicy peanut sauce with cinnamon and chilli is beautifully warming and gives the greens a lovely crunchy texture and a wonderful sweet and tart flavour. The combination of healthy fats in the sauce with rich roasted greens aids absorption of the nutrients. This sauce is so delicious and the flavour gets better with age, so make a double batch to keep in a sealed jar in the fridge, for another use.

2 tbsp olive oil

300g Brussels sprouts, trimmed and halved

200g kale, stems removed, leaves shredded

For the peanut sauce

50ml olive oil

60g unsalted roasted peanuts, very finely chopped (you can do this in a food processor to save time)

2 garlic cloves, grated

2 tsp sesame seeds

2 tbsp tamari or **soy sauce**

1 tbsp sherry vinegar or **red wine vinegar**

10g soft light brown sugar

1 tsp chilli flakes

1 tsp toasted sesame oil

Pinch of ground cinnamon

Substitutions

Sherry vinegar: apple cider vinegar or balsamic vinegar

Preheat the oven to 220ºC fan.

Pour the oil into a large roasting tin and set it on the middle shelf of the oven to heat for a few minutes. Put the sprouts in the roasting tin, cut-side down, season with a pinch of salt and roast for 20 minutes until deeply charred and beginning to soften.

Stir in the kale and return to the oven for 6 to 7 minutes. (Depending on the size of your tray, you may need to use two trays to make sure they are not overcrowded and the greens crisp up nicely.)

Meanwhile, to make the sauce, heat the olive oil in a small saucepan over a medium heat, add the peanuts and cook for 2 to 3 minutes until golden. Remove from the heat and add the garlic and sesame seeds. Let everything bubble up for 1 minute then stir in the remaining ingredients. Keep stirring until the sugar has dissolved, then pour into a bowl and leave to cool.

Pour the sauce over the vegetables, toss to coat, then spoon into bowls and serve.

FENNEL & BLACK BEAN SALAD WITH CHIMICHURRI

Serves 2

Prep time: 15 minutes
Cook time: 15 minutes

This fennel salad is fresh, vibrant and filling thanks to the fibre and protein-rich black beans. It will also work well with poached chicken or leftover cooked meats. Traditionally, this chimichurri is made with fresh parsley, but you can use other soft herbs such as mint and coriander.

For the salad

1 x 400g can black beans, drained and rinsed

60g walnuts, roughly chopped

1 small fennel bulb, thinly sliced (preferably with a mandolin)

300g tomatoes, roughly chopped

For the chimichurri

75ml olive oil

2 tbsp red wine vinegar

1 red chilli, finely chopped

1 garlic clove, grated

1 tsp dried oregano

Large bunch of parsley (50g), finely chopped

Substitutions

Fennel: chicory or red cabbage

Black beans: haricot beans, pinto beans or chickpeas

Parsley: mint or coriander

Preheat the oven to 200°C fan.

Spread the beans and walnuts out on separate halves of a baking tray in an even layer and roast for 15 minutes until the nuts are toasted and the beans are dry and starting to crack and blister. Make sure the walnuts do not burn; remove them earlier from the oven if necessary.

Leave to cool to room temperature.

Meanwhile, mix the chimichurri ingredients together in a large bowl, with a pinch of salt.

Place the fennel in a large salad bowl and massage for 1 minute using your hands to soften. Add the remaining ingredients to the bowl and toss the chimichurri through to coat. Check the seasoning and serve.

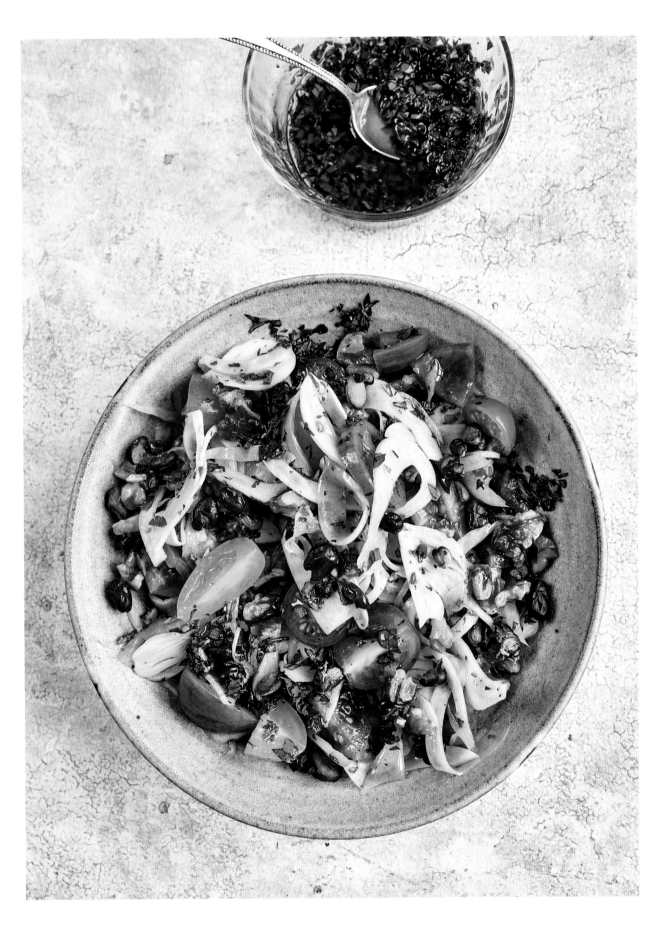

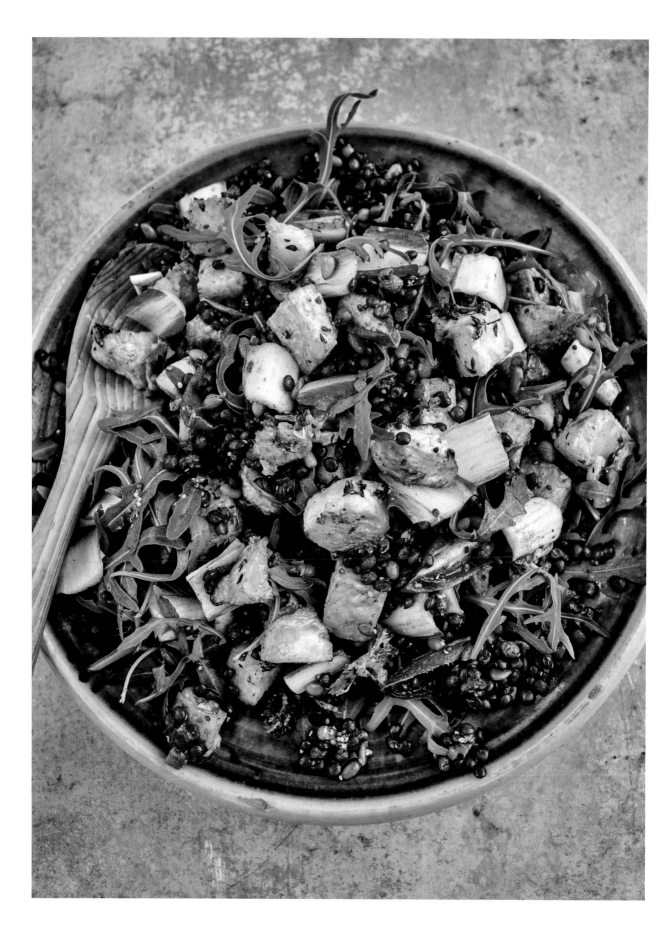

ROAST CELERIAC SALAD WITH RADICCHIO

Serves 2 generously

Prep time: 15 minutes
Cook time: 35 minutes

This simple dish makes use of a vegetable everyone struggles to think of what to do with. I wanted to make the humble celeriac the centrepiece here, with its distinctive flavour mellowed by the sweet roasted garlic and Parmesan umami.

300g celeriac, peeled and cut into 2cm cubes

2 tbsp extra virgin olive oil, plus a drizzle

2 garlic cloves, grated

40g Parmesan, **pecorino** or **vegetarian/vegan Italian hard cheese**, finely grated

4 sprigs of thyme, leaves only

250g cooked Puy lentils

30g pine nuts

2 tbsp red wine vinegar

1 tbsp wholegrain mustard

1 tbsp capers

100g red chicory or **radicchio**, roughly chopped

100g rocket

Preheat the oven to 200°C fan, and preheat a roasting tin for a few minutes.

Tip the celeriac into the tin, drizzle with olive oil and season with a little salt and pepper. Roast for 20 minutes. Remove from the oven and toss through the garlic, cheese and thyme and roast for a further 10 minutes or until the celeriac is a deep golden.

Remove from the oven and stir in the lentils, pine nuts, vinegar, mustard and capers, with a drizzle more extra virgin olive oil.

Toss through the leaves to bring in all the flavour, then pile them into a mound on a large serving platter. Check the seasoning and serve.

Substitutions

Celeriac: sweet potato, parsnips or turnips

Pine nuts: flaked almonds, sunflower seeds or pumpkin seeds

SHREDDED CABBAGE & CHESTNUT SALAD WITH KIMCHI

Serves 2

Prep time: 20 minutes
Cook time: 10 minutes

I love using the sharp and tangy kimchi juice as a dressing to perk up simple salad ingredients. The crispy chestnuts work really well to give body and texture to this salad and the flavour combination of heat and umami works well with the fresh raw greens. Use the substitutions suggested below to make this salad entirely plant based.

½ **small white cabbage** (200g), finely shredded

2 **tbsp olive oil**

100g **chestnuts**, crumbled

160g **pak choi**, finely shredded

100g **baby tomatoes**, halved

2 **tbsp kimchi**, finely chopped

For the dressing

3 **tbsp kimchi juice** (from the packet or jar)

2 **tsp fish sauce** (optional)

1 **tbsp gochujang** or **sriracha**

2 **tbsp toasted sesame oil**

20g **toasted sesame seeds**

20g **fresh ginger**, grated

1 **lemongrass stalk**, tough outer leaves discarded, grated

Whisk all the dressing ingredients together in a large bowl.

Add the cabbage to the bowl with the dressing, massage for 2 to 3 minutes, using your hands, until softened and set aside.

Heat the oil in a large frying pan over a high heat, add the chestnuts and stir-fry for 5 minutes until crisp and golden, then set aside.

Add the pak choi, tomatoes, kimchi and chestnuts to the bowl with the white cabbage and toss to combine. Check the seasoning and serve.

Substitutions

Fish sauce: mushroom sauce or tamari

Gochujang: sriracha or red chilli sauce

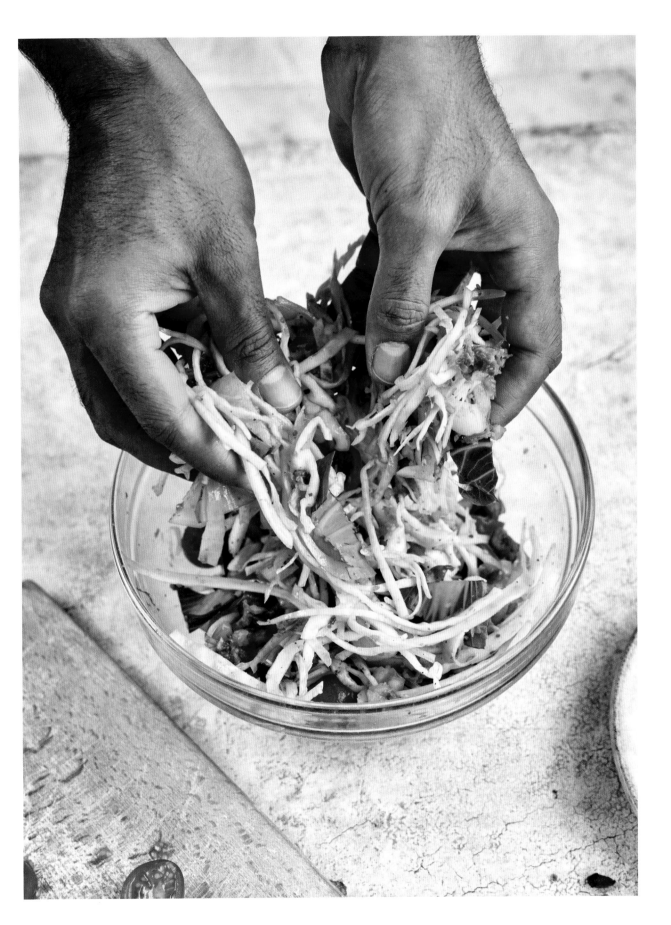

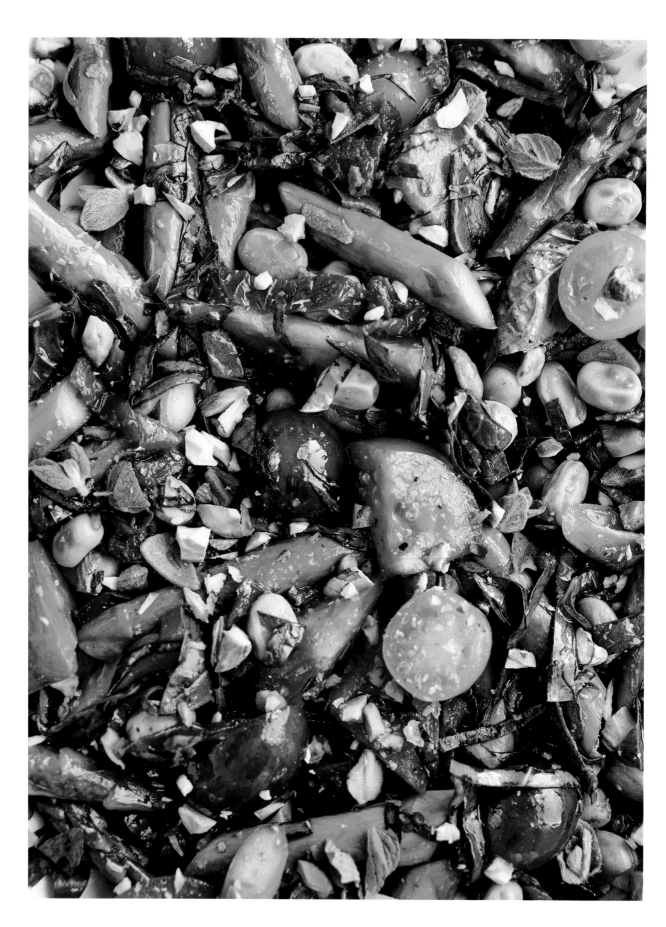

SPRING SAUTÉ

Serves 2 generously

Prep time: 15 minutes
Cook time: 15 minutes

This green sauté has a vibrant flavour with a vinegary kick from the sharp dressing and an umami saltiness from the sun-dried tomatoes. It's a perfect collection of spring ingredients to add variety to your weekly diet, and the produce does most of the work.

100g baby leaf spinach, finely sliced

10g basil leaves, roughly torn

200g heritage tomatoes, roughly chopped

200g podded broad beans (fresh or frozen, also see Note below)

200g asparagus spears, roughly chopped into 3cm lengths

2 tbsp olive oil

20g sun-dried tomatoes in oil, roughly chopped

2 garlic cloves, sliced

30g pistachios, toasted and very finely chopped

1 lemon, cut into wedges, to serve

For the dressing

2 tbsp extra virgin olive oil

Finely grated zest and **juice of ½ lemon**

1 tsp pomegranate molasses

4 sprigs of oregano, leaves only (or 2 tsp dried oregano)

1 tsp cayenne pepper or **smoked paprika**

Whisk the dressing ingredients together in a large bowl, seasoning to taste. Add the spinach, basil and fresh tomatoes, and set aside.

Bring a large saucepan of salted water to the boil. Drop the broad beans into the pan, cook for 3 minutes then add the asparagus. Cook for a further 2 minutes, then drain. (If using frozen broad beans, defrost them thoroughly then cook together with the asparagus for 2 minutes only.)

Add the olive oil to a large sauté pan, along with a tablespoon of the sun-dried tomato oil. Add the garlic to the pan and cook for 2 to 3 minutes until starting to brown. Add the broad beans, asparagus and sun-dried tomatoes and sauté for 4 to 5 minutes.

Tip the sautéed greens into the salad bowl with the other ingredients and use tongs to mix everything together so the spinach gently wilts in the residual heat of the greens. Serve sprinkled with the chopped pistachios and lemon wedges.

Note

I reserve the cooking water from the broad beans to enjoy as a green-infused drink. Add a squeeze of lemon and a pinch of salt for a nourishing hot tonic.

STICKY TANGY GREEN BEANS

Serves 4 as a side

Prep time: 15 minutes
Cook time: 10 minutes

This sticky dressing is divine. I'm sure you will find many uses for it in your kitchen, but my favourite way is to simply drizzle it over crisp sugar snap peas and delicious green beans blanched in hot water.

300g sugar snap peas, finely sliced

300g green beans, roughly chopped into 3cm pieces

300g cooked brown lentils

1 small red pepper (120g), deseeded and finely chopped

10g coriander, leaves and stalks finely chopped

10g mint, leaves only, finely chopped

For the dressing

2 tsp tamarind paste

4 tbsp date molasses or **coconut sugar**

4 tbsp black vinegar or **sherry vinegar**

4 tbsp tamari or **soy sauce**

1 garlic clove, grated

Juice of 1 lime

Mix the dressing ingredients in a pan over a medium heat and bring to a gentle simmer. Cook for 8 minutes or until reduced to a thick, sticky mixture that thickly coats the back of a spoon.

Meanwhile, blanch the sugar snaps and green beans in a large pan of boiling water for 3 minutes, then drain thoroughly.

Toss onto a large platter with the lentils and red pepper, drizzle the sticky dressing over the top and carefully toss through with tongs. Scatter over the herbs and serve.

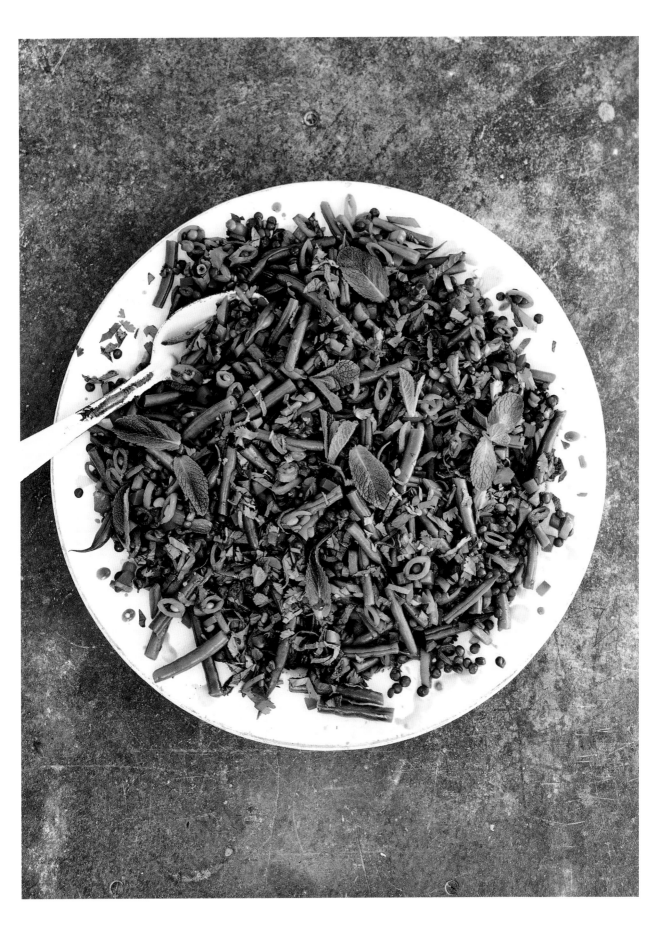

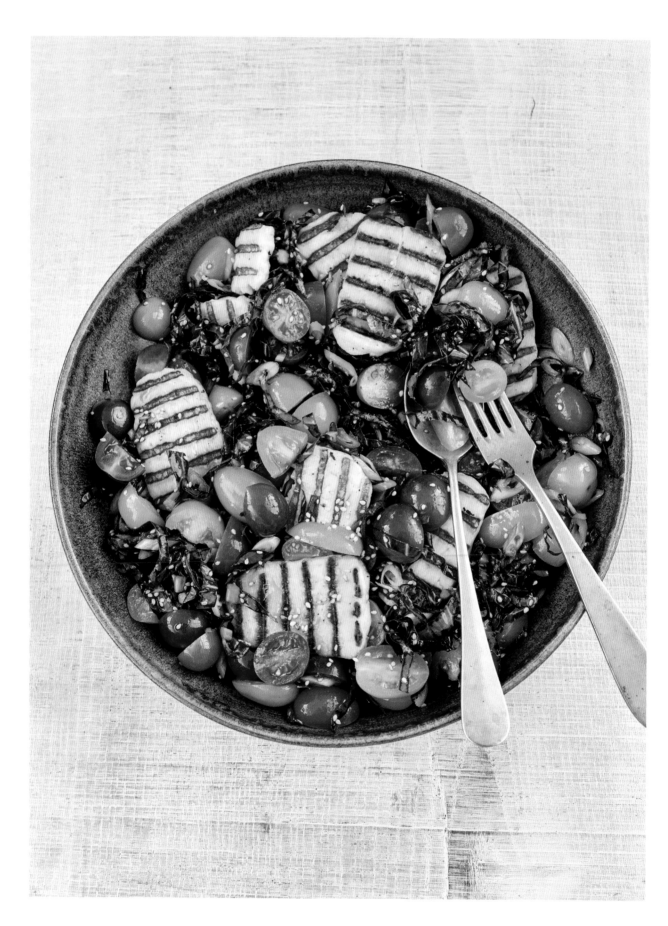

SWEET & SHARP TOMATO & HALLOUMI SALAD

Serves 4 as a side salad

Prep time: 15 minutes, plus marinating
Cook time: 5 minutes

This is a beautifully simple side dish with a lovely salty yet clean-tasting dressing that sits in the background and lifts the natural sweetness of fresh tomatoes. Use heritage tomatoes if you can get hold of them in season – they make a world of difference with this dressing, and taste gorgeous.

100g spring greens, finely shredded

400g mixed tomatoes, smaller ones halved, larger ones cut into bite-sized chunks

250g halloumi, sliced 1cm thick

50g spring onions, sliced on an angle

For the dressing

25ml rice vinegar

25ml tamari or **soy sauce**

40ml toasted sesame oil

2 garlic cloves, grated

½ tsp chilli flakes

50g toasted sesame seeds

Whisk the dressing ingredients together in a large salad bowl. Add the spring greens to the bowl with a pinch of salt. Using your hands, massage the dressing into the greens for a minute, then add the tomatoes and leave to marinate in the mixture. (Marinating for 30 minutes in the fridge is ideal, but if you don't have time then don't worry.)

Cook the halloumi slices in a sauté pan or griddle pan for 3 to 4 minutes on each side until nicely golden.

Toss the halloumi and spring onions through the tomatoes and greens in the bowl and serve.

Substitutions

Halloumi: silken tofu cut into cubes for a vegan alternative

Rice vinegar: balsamic vinegar or pomegranate vinegar

Sesame seeds: unsalted roasted peanuts, finely chopped or sunflower seeds, lightly crushed or simply omit

WATERCRESS & LENTIL SALAD WITH MUSHROOMS & OLIVES

Serves 2

Prep time: 10 minutes
Cook time: 30 minutes

Meaty charred mushrooms, citrus acidity and sweet shallots are the core flavours of this simple dish that is super-easy to prepare. The robust lentils and peppery rocket take on the flavours well and it's packed with nutrition to help you maintain a diverse and interesting range of plants in your diet.

300g mixed mushrooms (I use shiitake and oyster), sliced

3 tbsp olive oil, plus extra to serve

160g shallots, thinly sliced lengthways

2 garlic cloves, grated

60g pistachios, roughly chopped

30g pitted Kalamata olives, roughly chopped

Finely grated zest and **juice of ½ lemon**

200g cooked Puy lentils

5g tarragon, finely chopped

150g watercress, roughly torn

Substitutions

Puy lentils: white beans

Tarragon: parsley

Watercress: rocket

Heat a sauté pan or deep frying pan over a medium-high heat. Add the mushrooms without any oil and stir around the pan for 5 minutes to dry off their water content, then add half the oil and sauté for a further 5 to 6 minutes with some seasoning, stirring regularly, until deeply caramelised.

Transfer to a plate and set aside. Reduce the heat slightly, add the remaining oil then fry the shallots with some seasoning for 10 to 15 minutes until soft and caramelised.

Add the garlic and pistachios, fry for 3 to 4 minutes, then stir in the olives and lemon zest.

Add the lentils, return the mushrooms to the pan, then remove from the heat and stir through the lemon juice and tarragon.

Add to a large platter with the watercress and toss together, drizzle with extra olive oil and season to taste with a pinch of salt and pepper.

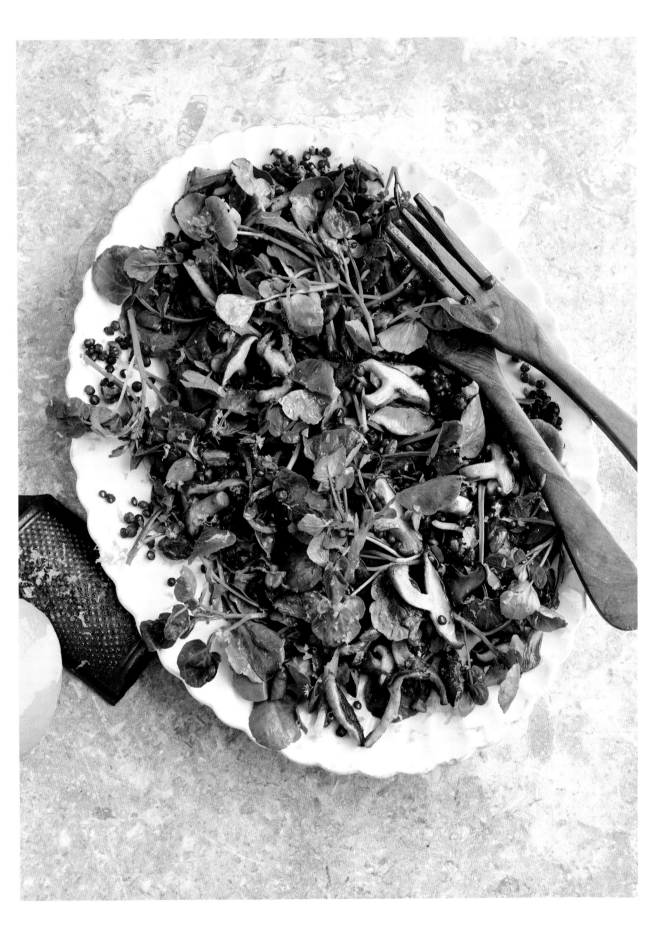

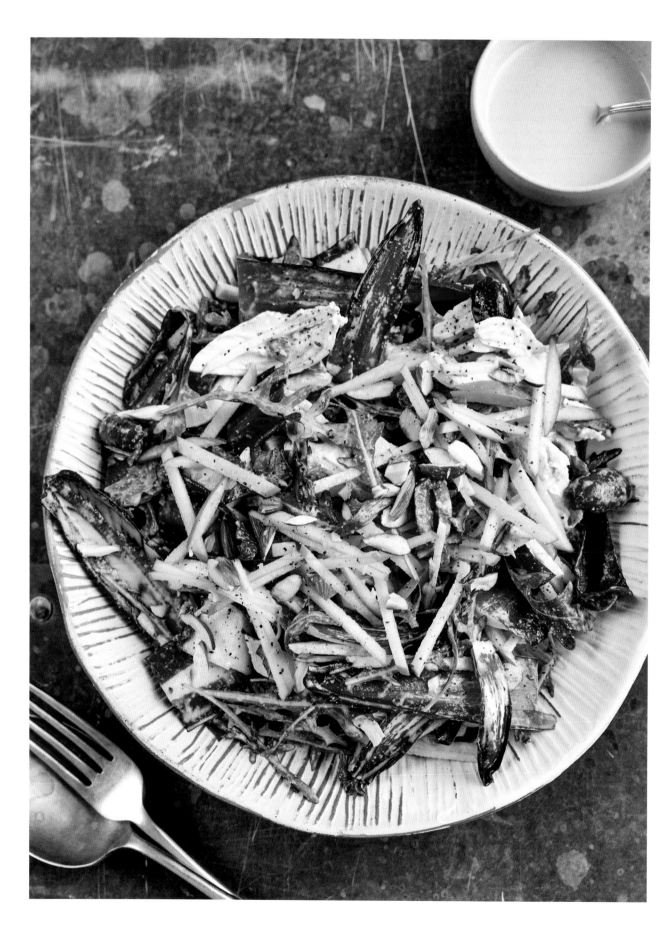

LEMON-POACHED CHICKEN SALAD WITH TAHINI DRESSING

Serves 2 generously

Prep time: 10 minutes
Cook time: 25 minutes

This simple chicken salad is a perfect collection of vibrant colours, flavours and good-quality storecupboard ingredients. The olive, pine nut and bitter leaves combination is a personal favourite of mine and is a wonderful way to get those plant chemical-rich ingredients into your diet.

Pared zest of 1 lemon

2 whole star anise

½ tsp black peppercorns

300g boneless, skinless chicken breasts

For the dressing

4 tbsp tahini

2 tbsp extra virgin olive oil

Juice of 1 lemon (use the zested lemon)

1 garlic clove, grated

For the salad

160g rocket, roughly chopped

160g red chicory or **radicchio**, chopped

1 green apple, cored and julienned

60g pitted Kalamata olives, torn

60g toasted almonds, chopped

Small bunch of tarragon (20g), leaves chopped

Using a vegetable peeler, pare the zest of the lemon into a large saucepan with the star anise, peppercorns and a pinch of salt, then pour over 800ml water.

Bring the water to the boil and add the chicken breasts. Reduce to a gentle simmer, then cover with a lid and cook gently for 10 to 12 minutes. Lift the chicken out of the pan and set aside to rest before slicing thinly.

Spoon 75ml of the chicken poaching liquid into a large bowl and whisk in the tahini, oil, lemon juice, garlic and some salt and pepper, until you have a smooth sauce.

Add the rocket, chicory, apple, olives, almonds and tarragon to a bowl. Add the sliced chicken, then drizzle over the dressing and toss to coat. Check the seasoning and serve.

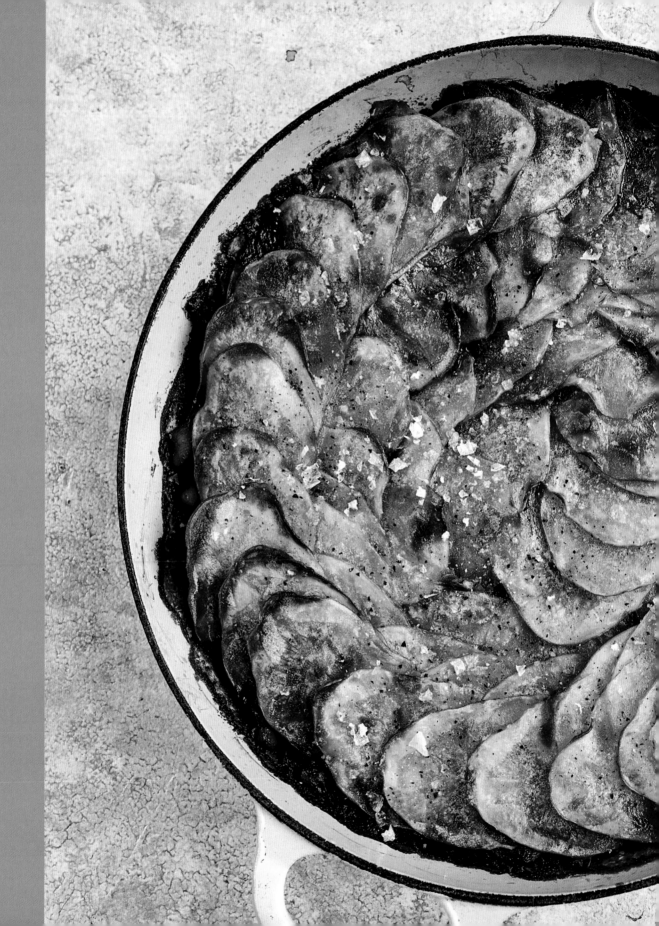

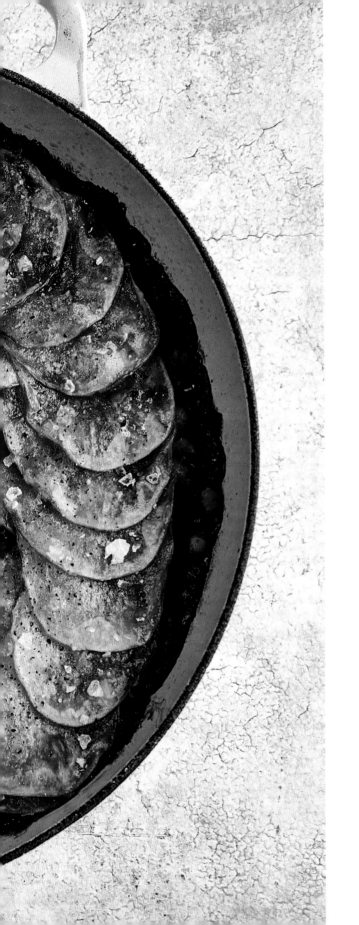

CASSEROLES

CHESTNUT & WHITE BEAN STEW WITH CAVOLO NERO

Serves 2

Prep time: 15 minutes
Cook time: 15 minutes

This is my ultimate comfort food: creamy, nutty beans, a hug of sage and hint of lemon. A great winter meal that's super quick and simple with minimal ingredients. This was one of my recipe testers' most popular dishes – it won't disappoint.

2 tbsp **extra virgin olive oil**

180g **cooked chestnuts**, roughly crumbled

3 **garlic cloves**, grated

8 **sage leaves**, finely chopped

Finely grated zest of 1 lemon and **a squeeze of juice**

2 tbsp **white miso paste** (gluten-free, if neceassary)

500ml **vegetable stock**

1 x 400g can **cannellini beans**, drained and rinsed

200g **cavolo nero**, stems removed, leaves roughly chopped

25g **toasted hazelnuts**, chopped, to serve

Heat the oil in a lidded saucepan over a medium heat, add the chestnuts, garlic, sage and lemon zest and fry for 2 to 3 minutes.

Stir in the miso paste then add the stock and beans. Bring to a simmer then cover and cook for 5 minutes.

Stir in the cavolo nero, cover with a lid and cook for a further 3 to 4 minutes. Season with a pinch each of salt and pepper and add a squeeze of lemon juice.

Serve the beans in bowls, scattered with the toasted hazelnuts.

Substitutions

Cavolo nero: hispi cabbage

Roasted hazelnuts: plain nuts, blanched almonds, macadamia or pecans

Fresh sage leaves: 2 tsp dried sage, thyme or rosemary

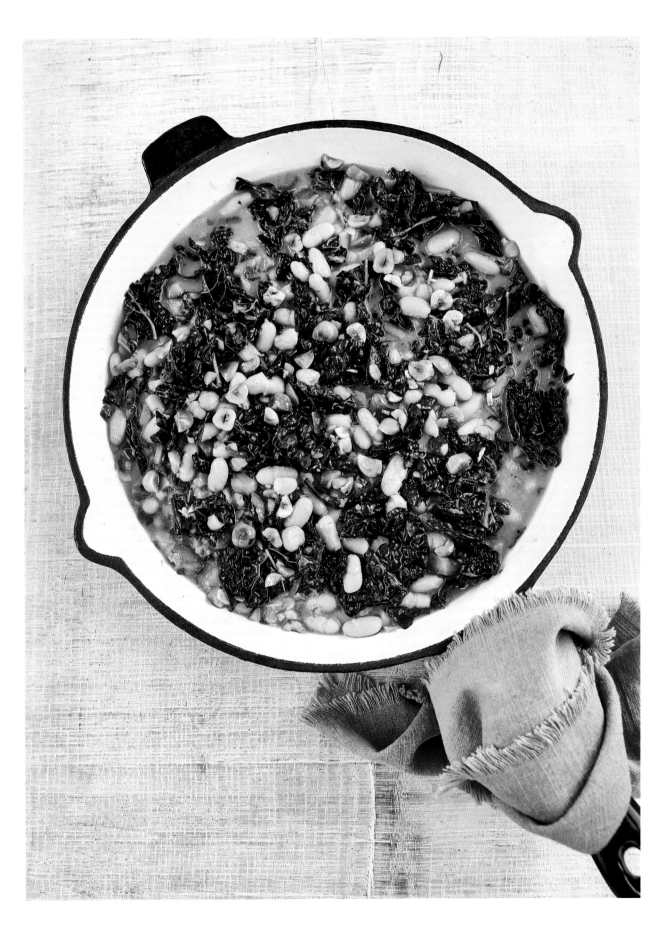

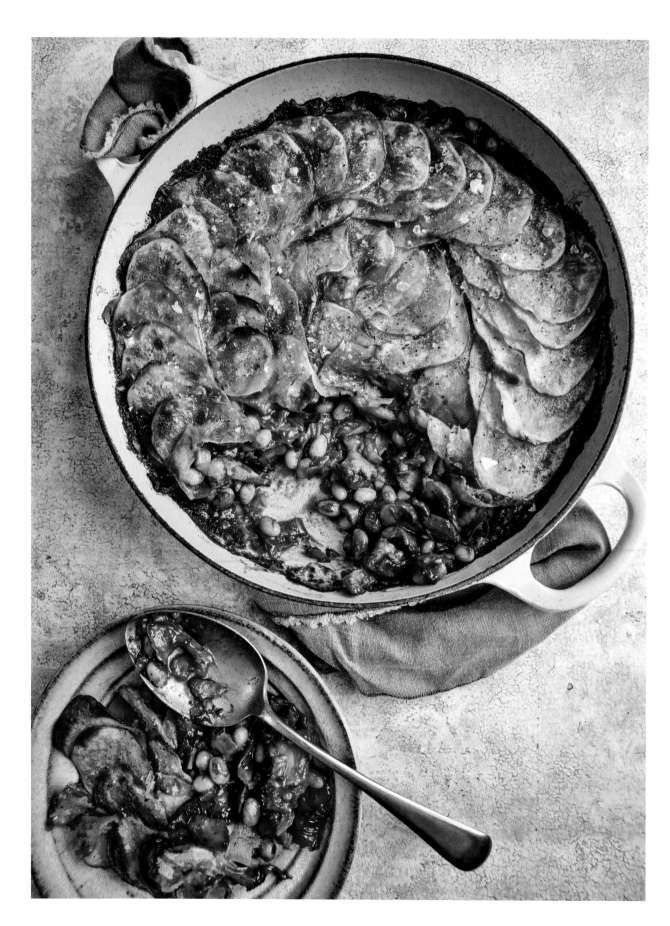

HARICOT BEAN CASSEROLE

Serves 4

Prep time: 25 minutes
Cook time: 50 minutes

This is a wintry comfort dish packed with three different types of prebiotic-rich vegetables that deliver a beautiful undertone of sweetness to the meal. The subtle aniseed flavour of tarragon with earthy oregano is also delicious, and the soy enriches the sauce with a gorgeous body of flavour.

3 tbsp olive oil, plus extra to drizzle

1 large red onion (180g), roughly chopped

400g leeks, roughly chopped

400g brown mushrooms, roughly chopped

1 tsp ground cinnamon

2 tsp dried oregano

2 tsp dried tarragon

1 tsp ground black pepper

1 vegetable stock cube, crumbled

1 x 400g can haricot beans, drained and rinsed

3 tbsp tamari or **soy sauce**

3 tbsp tomato purée

1 tbsp cornflour

400ml hot water

1 large white potato, scrubbed and left unpeeled, cut into thin (1–2mm) rounds with a mandolin

Preheat the oven to 200°C fan.

Heat the oil in a large flameproof casserole over a medium heat, add the onion, leeks and mushrooms, season with salt and sweat down for 15 minutes.

Add the remaining ingredients except the potato, stir until all the elements combine and bring to a gentle simmer for 5 minutes.

Place the potato slices on top in an overlapping layer, drizzle with olive oil and sprinkle generously with salt. Bake in the oven for 30 minutes until the potato is cooked and browned, and the mixture is bubbling away underneath. Leave to stand for 5 minutes before serving.

HERBY BEAN & ALMOND GRATIN

Prep time: 20 minutes
Cook time: 35 minutes

I love the ease and herb flavour of this dish. You can change up the dried herbs for whatever is in the cupboard. I always try to remind people that the beauty of dried herbs is concentrated flavour, but there is also evidence that they retain a lot of the beneficial plant chemicals that are found in fresh herbs too.

2 tbsp olive oil

160g cavolo nero, stems finely chopped, leaves shredded

160g spring greens, stems finely chopped, leaves shredded

Small bunch of spring onions (120g), chopped

6 garlic cloves, chopped

1 tsp chilli flakes

Sprig of rosemary, leaves chopped

1 x 400g can butter beans or **cannellini beans**, drained and rinsed

500ml vegetable stock

25g Parmesan or **vegetarian/ vegan Italian hard cheese**, finely grated

Finely grated zest of 1 lemon

For the topping

75g oats (gluten-free, if necessary)

60g ground almonds

25g Parmesan or **vegetarian/ vegan Italian hard cheese**, finely grated

1 tbsp olive oil

1 tsp dried oregano

1 tsp dried thyme

Preheat the oven to 200°C fan.

Heat the oil in a flameproof casserole over a medium heat. Put the chopped stems of the cavolo nero and spring greens into the casserole, add the spring onions, garlic and chilli flakes and fry for 6 minutes until softened and starting to caramelise. Stir in the shredded leaves, rosemary and beans, stirring carefully for a further 2 minutes.

Add the stock and simmer for 5 minutes, then add the Parmesan and lemon zest and season with salt and pepper. Cook for a further 2 minutes.

Meanwhile, combine the topping ingredients in a bowl, season with a pinch of salt and mix thoroughly.

Scatter the topping over the beans and vegetables in an even layer and drizzle with a little extra olive oil. Transfer to the oven and bake for 20 minutes until golden brown. Leave to stand for 5 minutes before serving.

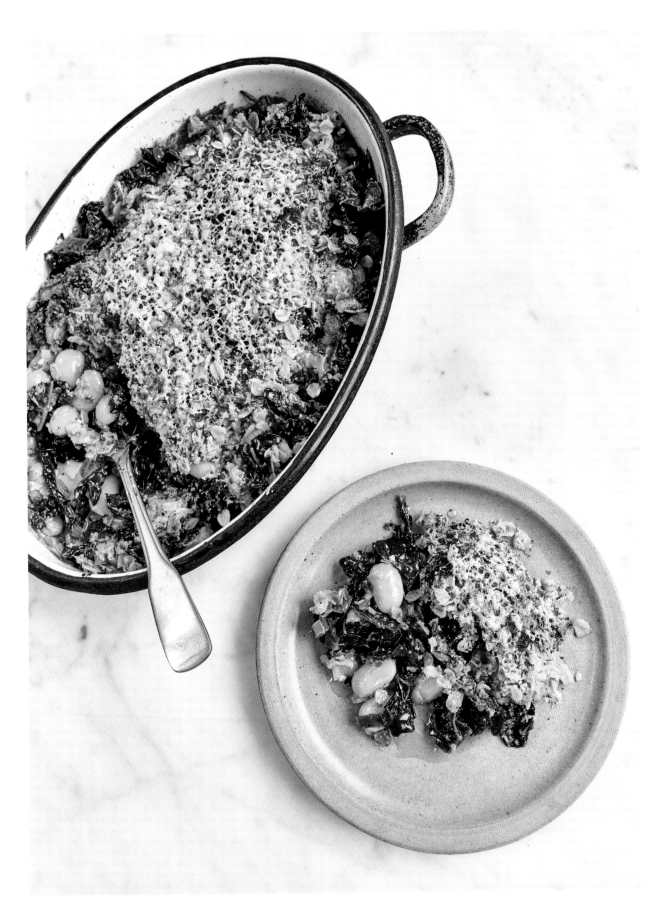

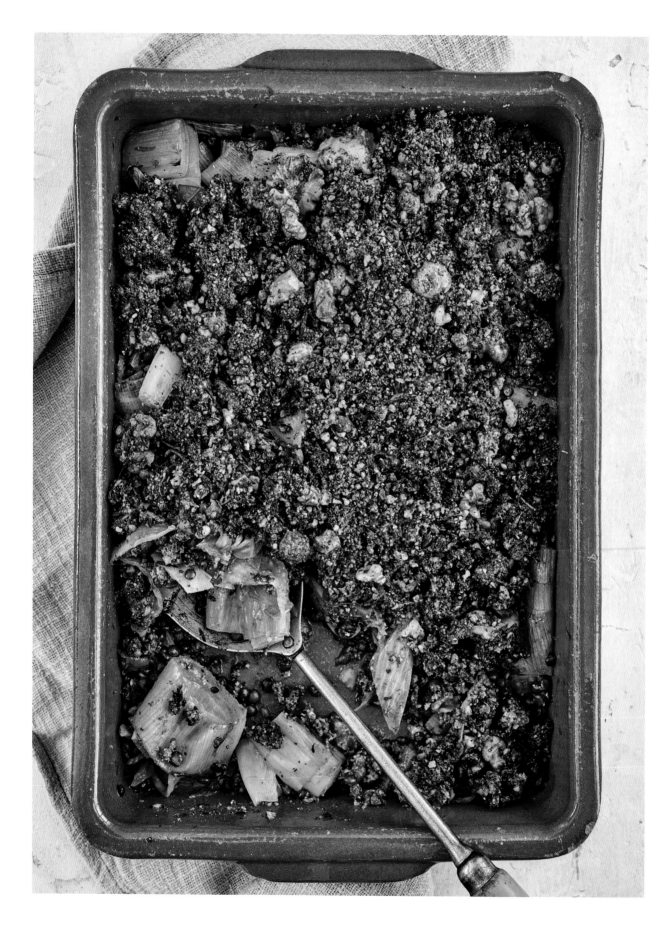

MUSHROOM & LEEK GRATIN

Serves 4

Prep time: 20 minutes
Cook time: 40 minutes

This easy family-style meal has a delicious depth of flavour from the dried mushrooms, and the walnuts deliver a lovely crumb for the topping. I've packed this with allium vegetables and Puy lentils that give a body to this casserole.

3 tbsp olive oil

2 leeks (300g), sliced into 2cm rounds

1 large fennel bulb (300g), thinly sliced

3 garlic cloves, grated

400g tomatoes, diced

400g cooked Puy lentils

100ml hot water

For the topping

50g dried mushrooms

100g walnuts

30g Parmesan or **vegetarian/ vegan Italian hard cheese**, finely grated

Pinch of chilli flakes

100ml hot water

Note

Dried mushrooms can be a bit gritty, so rinse them quickly in cold water and dry on kitchen paper before using.

Preheat the oven to 200°C fan.

Heat the oil in a flameproof lidded casserole over a medium heat, add the leeks and fennel and fry for 8 minutes until softened and starting to caramelise.

Add the garlic, fry for 1 minute, then add the tomatoes. Cover and cook for 10 minutes, stirring occasionally, until the tomatoes have broken down and the leeks are soft.

Meanwhile, put the dried mushrooms into a food processor and blend to a fine crumb. Add the walnuts, Parmesan and chilli flakes and pulse until coarsely chopped. With the motor running, gradually add the hot water; the mixture should resemble wet sand.

Stir the lentils into the vegetables along with the hot water, season with a pinch of salt and pepper then top with the mushroom and walnut crumb.

Transfer to the oven and bake for 15 minutes until the top is crisp and the sauce is bubbling at the edges. Leave to stand for 5 minutes before serving.

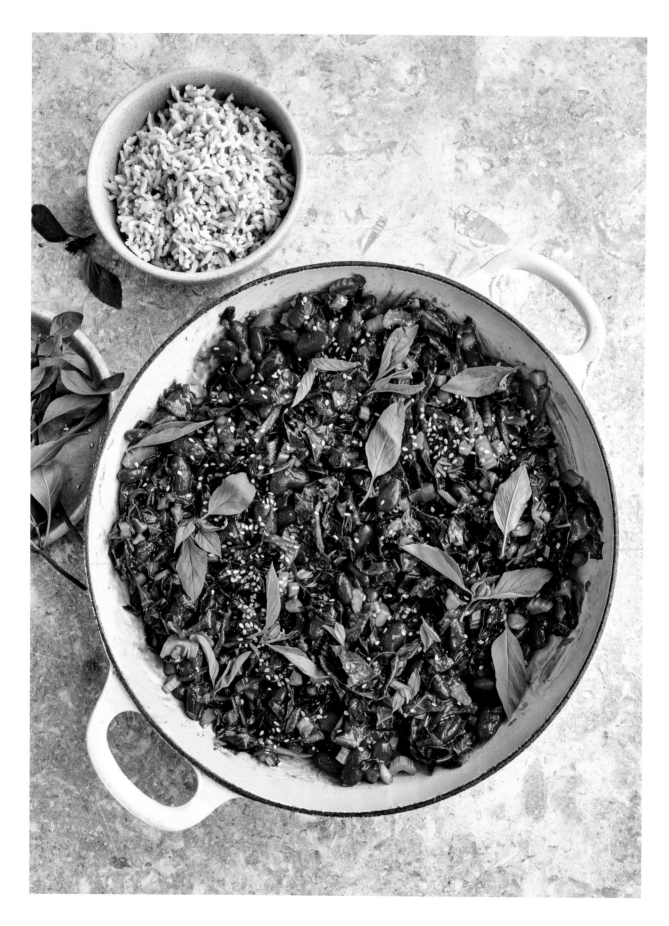

RED BEANS IN SWEET SPICY SAUCE

Serves 2 generously

Prep time: 20 minutes
Cook time: 40 minutes

This is hot, spicy, crunchy and gingery all at the same time, and the results are delicious and moreish. The celery delivers a slight crunch, which goes well with the fiery gochujang and beans. It will be a hit.

2 tbsp olive oil

1 large red onion (160g), sliced

8 garlic cloves, grated

1 whole star anise

20g fresh ginger, cut into thin matchsticks or grated

50ml tamari or soy sauce

300ml vegetable stock

2 tbsp mirin

2 tbsp tomato purée

1 tbsp gochujang or any chilli paste

1 tbsp brown sugar

1 tbsp cornflour

1 x 400g can red beans, drained and rinsed

200g celery, finely chopped

150g spring greens, stems removed, very finely chopped

To serve (optional)

150g cooked short-grain brown rice

10g sesame seeds

1 tsp sesame oil

10g Thai basil, torn

Heat the olive oil in a saucepan over a medium heat, add the onion and sauté for 8 minutes, then add the garlic, star anise and ginger, and cook for a further 3 minutes.

Pour in the tamari or soy sauce, stock and mirin, add the tomato purée, gochujang, sugar and cornflour, and bring to a simmer.

Cook for 20 minutes until thickened (you may need to add a splash of water if it gets too dry), then add the red beans, celery and spring greens and cook for a further 5 minutes until the greens have wilted. Season to taste.

Serve, if you like, with cooked brown rice and topped with sesame seeds, sesame oil and Thai basil leaves.

SPANISH-STYLE BLACK OLIVE, ALMOND & PINTO BEANS

Serves 4

Prep time: 20 minutes
Cook time: 35 minutes

The sweet smell of frying garlic and onions always reminds me of Spain and their wonderful rich cuisine full of yellow and deep red colours. This dish brings out the natural sweetness of allium vegetables with cinnamon, combined with the smoky heat of paprika and the saltiness of olive that makes for a well-rounded showstopping dish.

3 tbsp extra virgin olive oil

1 large red onion (180g), diced

300g leeks, sliced into half-moons

200g new potatoes, scrubbed and quartered

1–2 fresh red jalapeños or regular red chilli, sliced

6 garlic cloves, sliced

2 tbsp tomato purée

120g roasted almonds, roughly chopped (skin on is fine)

2 tsp ground cinnamon or 1 cinnamon stick

50g pitted black olives, sliced

2–3 tsp smoked paprika

600g tomatoes, roughly chopped

300ml hot water

1 x 400g can pinto beans, drained and rinsed

300g asparagus spears, halved lengthways if thick

10g chives, finely chopped

Heat the oil in a large flameproof casserole over a medium heat. Add the onion, leeks and potatoes and sauté for 6 to 7 minutes, then add the chilli and garlic and cook for a further 2 minutes. Make sure you season well.

Add the tomato purée, almonds, cinnamon, olives and paprika and stir for 1 minute before adding the tomatoes and hot water.

Bring to a simmer, cover and cook for 15 to 20 minutes until the potatoes have softened. Stir in the beans, place the asparagus stems on top and cover for a further 5 minutes until the asparagus is cooked and the potatoes are soft.

Remove the cinnamon stick, if necessary, and garnish the finished dish with the chopped chives before serving.

Substitutions

Fresh tomatoes: 2 x 400g cans chopped tomatoes

Asparagus: Tenderstem broccoli, runner beans or sugar snap peas

Pinto beans: borlotti beans or haricot beans

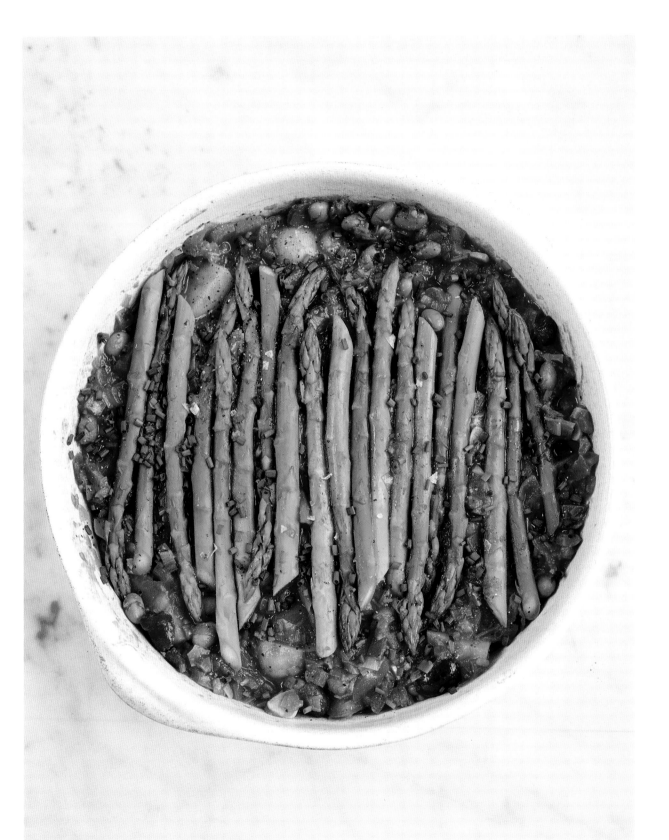

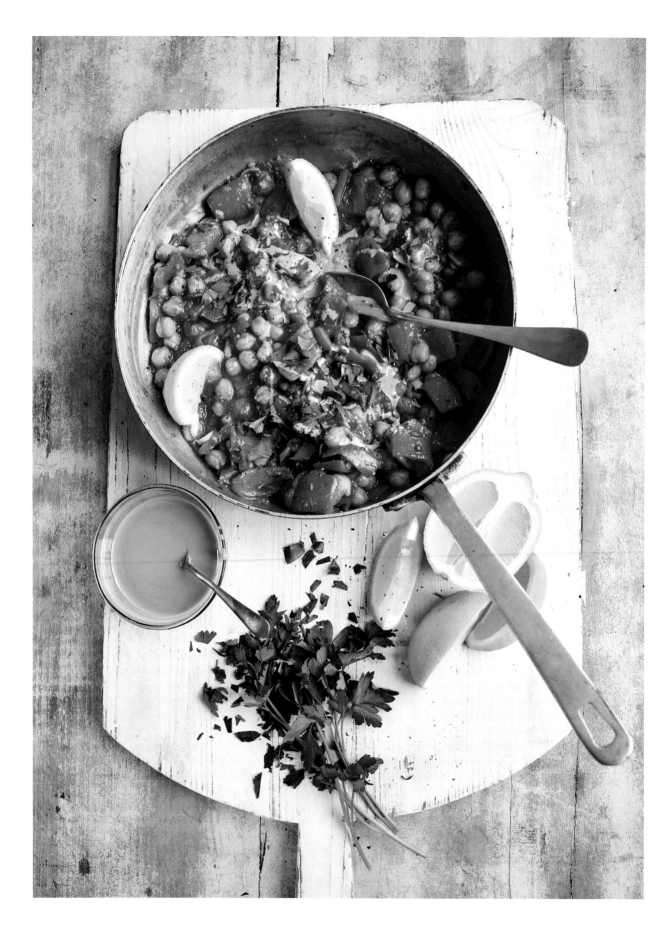

TUNISIAN-STYLE CHICKPEAS

Serves 2

Prep time: 10 minutes
Cook time: 30 minutes

This dish is brimming with spices, packed with flavour and delivers a wholesome and gorgeous meal with all the elements of an amazing dish that you will want to cook again and again. The peppers infused with all those spices give a beautiful warmth to the chickpeas that are packed with wholesome fibre.

3 tbsp **extra virgin olive oil**

2–3 **red romano peppers** (200g), deseeded and roughly chopped

1 tsp **fennel seeds**

1 tsp **caraway seeds**

1 tsp **cumin seeds**

1 tsp **coriander seeds**

3 **garlic cloves**, sliced

250g **tomatoes**, chopped

1 tbsp **tomato purée**

2 tsp **maple syrup** or **honey**

1 tbsp **harissa paste**, or to taste

1 **vegetable stock cube**

150ml **hot water**

1 x 400g **can chickpeas**, drained and rinsed

To serve

Large bunch of parsley (50g), roughly chopped

2 tbsp **tahini**

1 **lemon**, cut into wedges

Heat the oil in a wide flameproof casserole over a medium heat. Add the peppers with some seasoning, and cook gently for 5 to 6 minutes to soften. Add all the whole spices and garlic and cook for a further 1 minute to perfume the peppers and oil.

Add the tomatoes and cook for a further 10 minutes, stirring regularly until they break down.

Stir through the tomato purée, honey and harissa, then crumble in the stock cube and add the hot water. Stir in the chickpeas and simmer gently for 10 minutes until thickened.

Serve sprinkled with parsley and with a swirl of tahini over the top, with lemon wedges on the side.

ONE-POT CHICKEN CACCIATORE

Serves 2

Prep time: 15 minutes
Cook time: 45 minutes

A wintry, sumptuous herby casserole dish with gorgeous Mediterranean flavours and plenty of vegetables to hit that plant diversity. I've added beans to give this more fibre, while the hits of acidity from the wine and lemon plus the saltiness from the olives make this a well-balanced dish that I guarantee you will love.

3 tbsp extra virgin olive oil

4 skinless, boneless chicken thighs (275g)

2 shallots, diced

3 celery sticks (175g), sliced

2 carrots (180g), sliced

3 garlic cloves, grated

2 sprigs of rosemary

2 tsp dried oregano

1 tsp chilli flakes

1 x 400g can cannellini beans, drained and rinsed

100g tomato purée

50ml dry white wine

75g pitted black olives, roughly torn

350ml chicken stock or vegetable stock

Small bunch of parsley, chopped

Juice of ½ lemon

Heat half of the oil in a flameproof casserole over a medium-high heat.

Season the chicken with salt and pepper then brown all over for 6 to 7 minutes. Remove from the pan and set aside.

Add the remaining oil to the pan then add the shallots, celery, carrots and garlic and fry gently for 10 minutes until softened.

Stir in the rosemary, oregano, chilli flakes, beans and tomato purée. Cook for 2 minutes then pour in the wine and let it bubble up. Cook for a couple of minutes to burn off the alcohol.

Return the chicken to the pan, add the olives and stock bring everything to a simmer, then cover with a lid and cook for 25 minutes.

Season with a little salt and pepper and stir in the parsley and lemon juice. Pick out the rosemary stalks and serve.

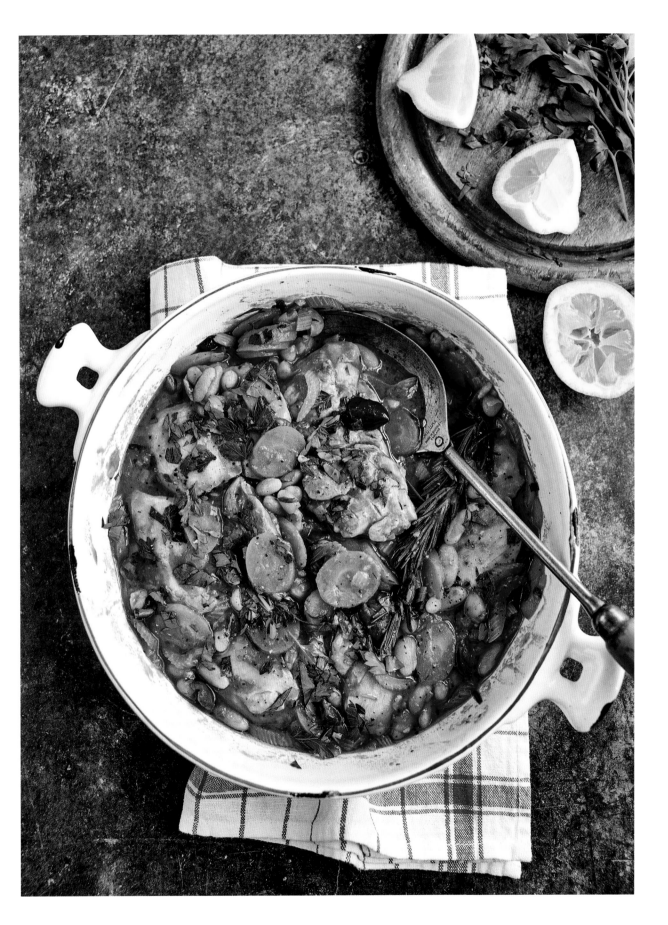

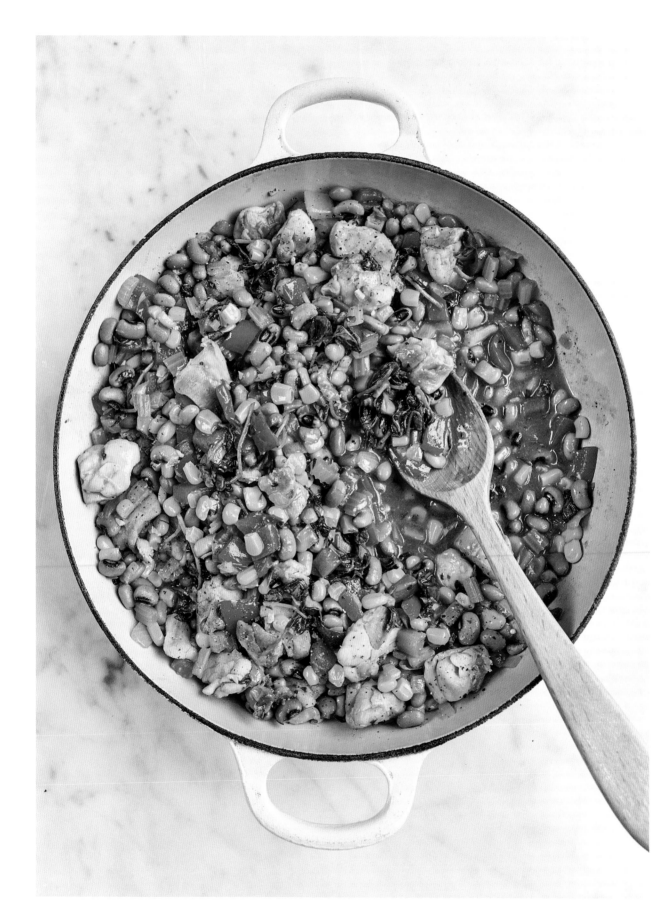

SPICY CHICKEN, SWEETCORN & BLACK-EYED BEANS

Serves 2 generously

Prep time: 15 minutes
Cook time: 30 minutes

This is my kind of store-cupboard ready meal. I always have these ingredients to hand to cook up whenever I'm in need of something delicious and nourishing. This works with and without the addition of chicken and the spices work wonderfully well. Make this plant based by simply omitting the chicken and adding another can of black-eyed beans.

2–3 tbsp olive oil

300g boneless, skinless chicken thighs, cut into 2cm chunks

1 red pepper (180g), deseeded and diced

1 onion (180g), peeled and diced

2 celery sticks (130g), diced

2 garlic cloves, diced

1 tsp cayenne pepper

1 tsp cumin seeds

½ tsp dried tarragon

1 bay leaf

200g sweetcorn (fresh, canned or frozen)

1 x 400g can black-eyed beans, drained and rinsed

1 vegetable stock cube

200ml hot water

50g watercress, roughly chopped

Heat 2 tablespoons of the oil in a large saucepan over a medium-high heat, add the chicken pieces, season and cook for 5 to 6 minutes, browning all over, then set aside on a plate.

Add a little more oil, then add the pepper, onion and celery and fry for 6 to 7 minutes, stirring regularly, until softened.

Add the garlic, spices and herbs and fry for 2 minutes, then return the chicken to the pan.

Tip in the sweetcorn and black-eye beans, crumble in the stock cube then pour in the hot water.

Cook, uncovered, over a medium heat for 15 minutes, stirring occasionally.

Stir in the watercress and season to taste with salt and pepper.

SIMPLE FISH STEW WITH GARLIC AIOLI

Serves 2 to 3

Prep time: 15 minutes
Cook time: 25 minutes

This is my take on a Mediterranean bourride, a dish similar to bouillabaisse but with a lighter taste and less heat. The celery, fennel and onion are a great fibre-rich base for the white fish, while the lemon and clove subtly perfume the stock. The simple aioli is a delicious addition to enrichen the stock with good-quality fats. A gorgeous summery dish that requires minimal cooking skill.

1 tbsp olive oil

200g celery, finely diced

1 small fennel bulb (200g), finely diced, fronds reserved

150g shallots or white onion, finely diced

1 tsp dried thyme

½ tsp fennel seeds

1 bay leaf

1 clove

3 strips of pared lemon zest

600ml fish stock or **vegetable stock**

400g skinless haddock, pollock or **monkfish**, cut into 4cm chunks

100g peas (podded if fresh or defrosted if frozen)

100g spinach, roughly chopped

For the garlic aioli

1 egg yolk

2 garlic cloves, grated

1 tsp wholegrain mustard

A squeeze of lemon juice

50ml extra virgin olive oil

To serve

Toasted sourdough (optional)

Lemon wedges

Make the garlic aioli in a small bowl by whisking together the egg yolk, garlic, mustard and lemon juice, with a pinch of seasoning. Gradually add the olive oil as you whisk, to emulsify the yolk. Set aside.

Heat a large, shallow flameproof casserole over a medium heat and add the olive oil, celery, fennel and shallots or onion, with a little seasoning. Sauté for 5 to 6 minutes until softened, then add the herbs, clove and lemon zest, and stir into the vegetables for a further 1 minute.

Add the stock, bring to a simmer for 2 minutes then turn the heat down low.

Add the fish chunks, cover with a lid and simmer for 5 minutes until the fish is cooked through. Use a slotted spoon to transfer the cooked fish to a plate.

Ladle a little of the cooking stock from your pan gradually into the bowl with the aioli and whisk until combined, then pour the aioli mixture into the pan and stir. It's very important to keep the pan over a low heat to ensure the mixture doesn't split.

Gently simmer to reduce the sauce for 7 to 8 minutes, stirring continuously with a whisk or spoon, until thickened.

Add the peas and spinach and let them wilt in the sauce for 2 minutes. Return the fish to the pan and serve with fennel fronds, toasted sourdough, and lemon wedges.

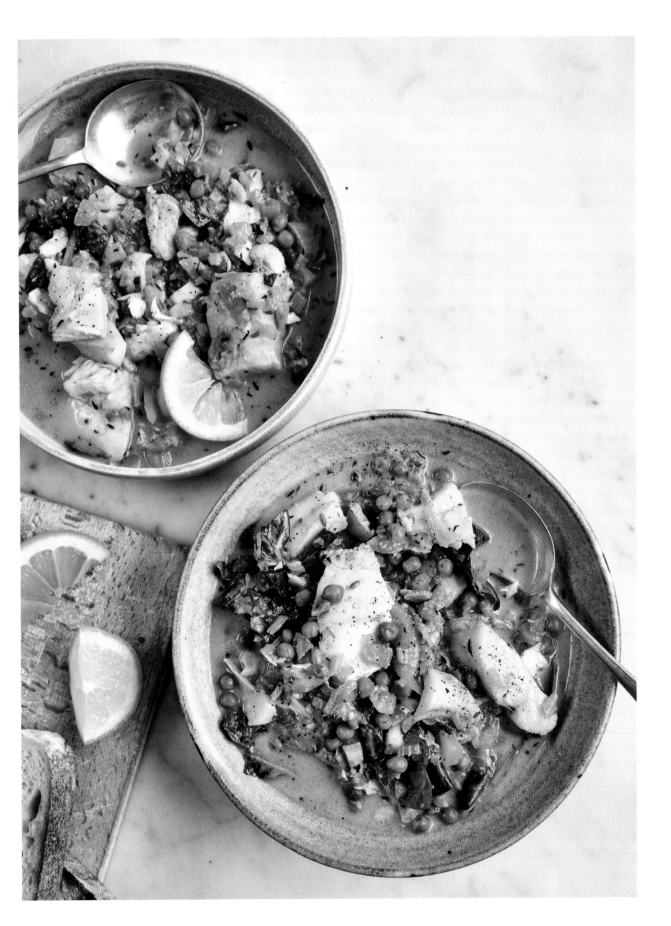

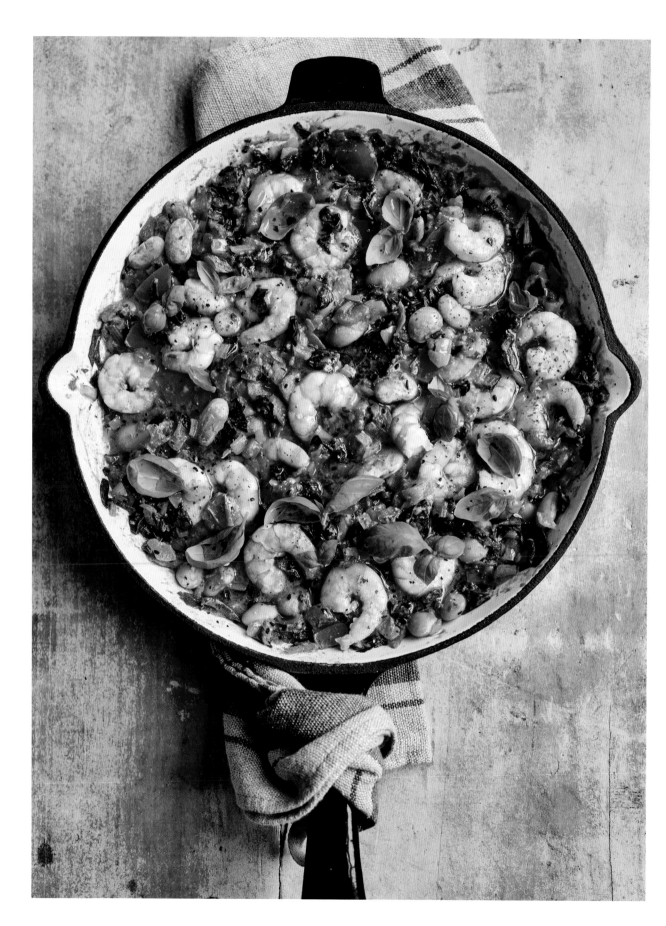

WHITE BEAN PRAWN SAGANAKI

GF

Serves 4

Prep time: 15 minutes
Cook time: 30 minutes

This dish will blow you away. The sauce is simple to make, but the flavours are intense, sweet and spicy. The caraway and nigella seeds lend an undertone of earthy flavours with the hum of garlic and kick of red chilli to counter. The greens and beans pack this with more vegetables, but the sauce is full of the good stuff too. You can easily make this vegetarian by simply substituting the prawns with more beans that have plenty of protein.

4 tbsp **extra virgin olive oil**

240g **white onion**, diced

5 **garlic cloves**, finely chopped

2 **red chillies**, finely chopped

2 tsp **caraway seeds**

2 tsp **nigella seeds**

2 tsp **dried oregano**

500g **tomatoes**, roughly chopped

2 tbsp **tomato purée**

2 tbsp **honey**

50g **feta**, crumbled

200g **chard** or **spinach leaves**, roughly chopped

20g **basil**, roughly chopped (reserve some leaves to garnish)

1 x 400g can **giant white beans** or **butter beans** (or any other white bean), drained and rinsed

200g **raw jumbo prawns**, shelled and deveined

Notes

For a smoother sauce, blend the chilli, garlic and onion in a small processor before cooking.

For even more flavour, toast the caraway and nigella seeds for 1–2 minutes and crush in a pestle and mortar before adding.

Preheat the grill to high.

Heat the oil in a flameproof casserole over a medium heat, add the onion and cook for 5 minutes until soft and translucent, then add the garlic, chilli and seasoning and cook for 2 minutes to colour and infuse their flavour.

Toss in the caraway and nigella seeds with the oregano and stir into the onions for 1 minute before adding the tomatoes, tomato purée, honey and feta. Cover and cook for 12 minutes until the tomatoes have fully broken down and the feta has melted into the sauce. Add a splash of water if it sticks to the bottom of the pan.

Uncover the pan and stir so that all the ingredients combine with the sauce, then add the green leaves and basil, reserving a few basil leaves to garnish, and stir for 2 to 3 minutes or until the greens have wilted.

Add the beans to the sauce and place the prawns on top. Simmer for 2 minutes then transfer to the grill for 4 minutes to finish cooking the prawns and caramelise the top of the dish.

Garnish with the reserved basil leaves and serve.

CAJUN-STYLE BEANS & PRAWNS

Serves 2 to 3

Prep time: 15 minutes
Cook time: 20 minutes

Lots of punchy herbs and spice pack an incredible amount of flavour into simple greens to make this prawn dish a memorable one. I serve this simply on its own, as the beans give a lot of body to the meal and taste absolutely amazing in the light sauce.

2 tbsp **extra virgin olive oil**

200g leeks, roughly chopped

200g shallot or **white onion**, diced

200g green pepper, deseeded and diced

4 garlic cloves, diced

1 bay leaf

1 tsp dried oregano

1 tsp dried thyme

1 tsp dried tarragon

½ tsp cayenne pepper

1 tsp smoked paprika

½ tsp ground black pepper

2 pared strips of zest and **juice of 1 lemon**

50ml dry white wine

2 tbsp Worcestershire sauce (optional)

300–350ml fish stock or **vegetable stock**

1 tsp cornflour

1 x 400g can haricot beans, drained and rinsed

400g raw jumbo prawns, shelled and deveined

Small bunch of parsley (20g), very finely chopped

Heat the oil in a shallow flameproof casserole over a medium heat and sauté the leeks, shallot or onion and green pepper, with seasoning, for 5 minutes.

Add the garlic, herbs, spices and lemon zest. Cook for a further 2 minutes to infuse their flavours.

Add the wine and half the lemon juice and let it bubble for a minute before adding the Worcestershire sauce, if using, stock and cornflour, stirring so all the ingredients come together, then tip in the beans.

Bring to a gentle simmer for a few minutes then add the prawns. When they turn pink, about 4 to 5 minutes, turn them all over in the dish and cook for a further 1 minute before taking off the heat, scattering with parsley and serving with more lemon juice.

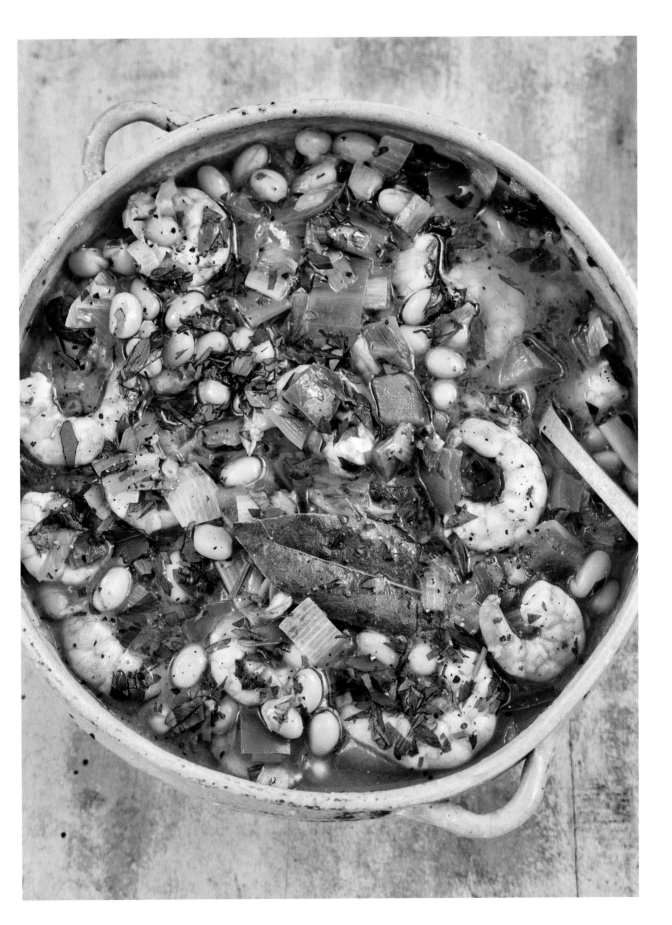

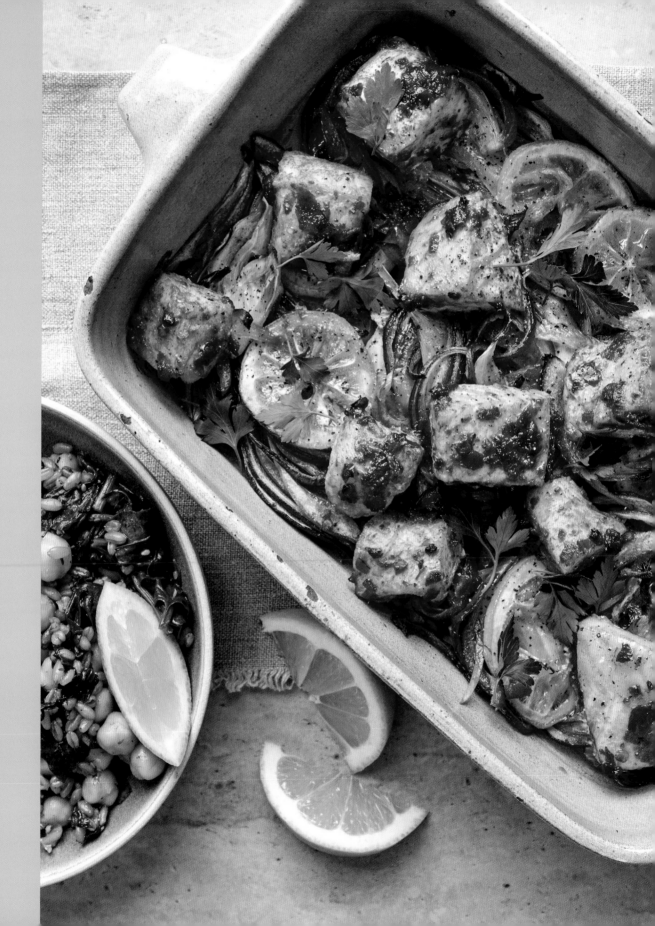

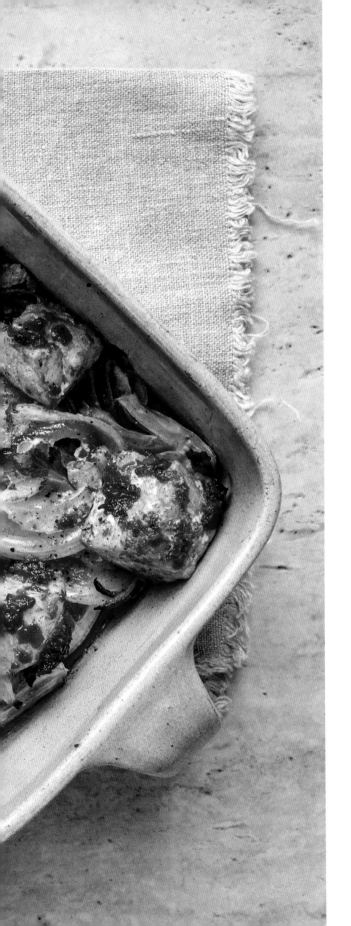

TRAYBAKES

AUBERGINE GREEN CURRY WITH SWEET PEANUT CRUMB

Serves 4

Prep time: 20 minutes
Cook time: 40 minutes

An earthy and satisfying curry with glorious Thai flavours that your family will love. I've simplified this recipe so you can easily make it in one tray, minimising the washing up and making it a perfect midweek meal packed with plant diversity, plant protein and plenty of anti-inflammatory benefits.

500g aubergines, cut into large cubes

400g tomatoes, quartered

3 tbsp coconut oil, melted

1 x 400ml can coconut milk

1 tbsp tamari or **soy sauce**

2–3 tbsp green curry paste (depending on your tolerance to spice)

1 x 400g can green lentils, drained and rinsed

300g tatsoi, halved lengthways

For the peanut crumb

40g unsalted roasted peanuts

1 tbsp brown sugar

½ tsp cracked black pepper

Substitutions

Aubergine: broccoli

Tatsoi: pak choi

Peanuts: sesame seeds

Preheat the oven to 200°C fan.

Tip the aubergines and tomatoes into a large roasting tin. Drizzle with the melted coconut oil, season with a large pinch of salt and cracked black pepper, then toss well to coat. Roast for 30 minutes until the aubergine is soft and tomatoes are broken down.

Meanwhile, combine the coconut milk, tamari or soy sauce and green curry paste in a bowl or jug.

Remove the roasting tin from the oven and tip in the lentils and coconut milk mixture. Stir the ingredients together until combined, then add the tatsoi to the sauce.

Return to the oven for a further 10 minutes until the greens are cooked and the sauce has reduced.

Meanwhile, to make the peanut crumb, pound the peanuts, sugar and pepper together with a pinch of salt in a pestle and mortar.

Remove the roasting tin from the oven and scatter the peanut crumb over the top to serve.

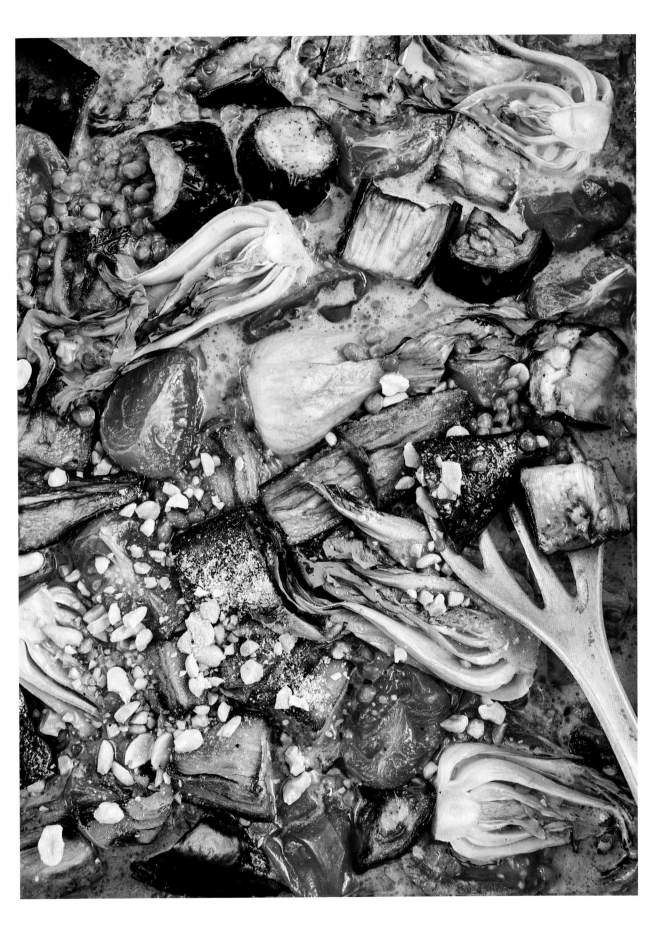

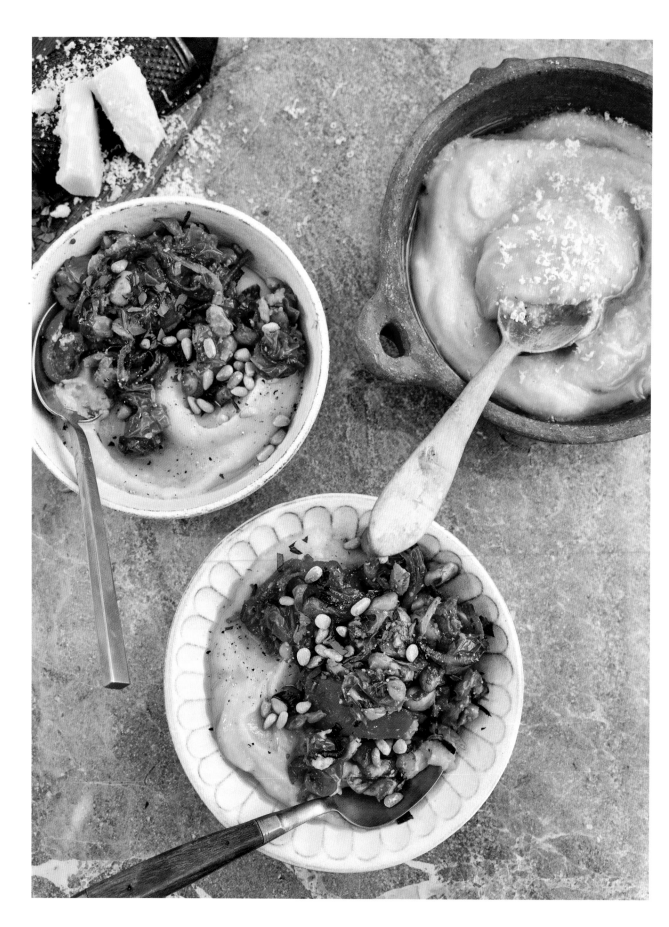

GARLICKY LEMON TOMATOES WITH QUICK POLENTA

Serves 2 generously

Prep time: 20 minutes
Cook time: 40 minutes

I usually crave robust, crunchy textures in my meals, but this sweet, tangy, garlicky dish on creamy, cheesy polenta is amazing. While it feels like indulgent comfort food, I've formulated it to contain ample vegetables. The polenta is a source of wholegrains and the combination is incredible. I've suggested some substitutions to make this vegan.

400g baby plum tomatoes, halved

1 red onion (160g), finely sliced

10 garlic cloves, lightly bashed

1 x 400g can borlotti beans, drained and rinsed

2 tbsp extra virgin olive oil

1 tbsp red wine vinegar

200g roasted red peppers, from a jar, drained and torn

2 tsp honey

2 tsp dried oregano

½–1 tsp chilli flakes

Finely grated zest of 1 lemon

Small bunch of parsley, chopped

2 tbsp toasted pine nuts or **hazelnuts,** to serve

For the polenta

700ml vegetable stock

120g instant polenta

2 tbsp extra virgin olive oil

2 tbsp finely grated Parmesan

Preheat the oven to 180°C fan. Place a large roasting tin in the oven for a few minutes to warm.

Tip the tomatoes, onion, garlic and beans into the roasting tin. Drizzle with the oil and vinegar, season with salt and pepper, then toss well to coat. Shake the tin until everything forms an even layer and roast for 20 minutes.

Remove the roasting tin from the oven and stir in the peppers, honey, oregano and chilli flakes. Return to the oven for a further 20 minutes, until sticky.

Meanwhile, bring the stock to the boil in a saucepan, whisk in the polenta then simmer gently for 8 to 10 minutes until thickened. Remove from the heat, beat in the oil and Parmesan, then season to taste.

Remove the roasting tray from the oven and grate the lemon zest over the veggies and beans.

Spoon the polenta into warm bowls and top with the roasted veggies and beans. Scatter the parsley and toasted pine nuts or hazelnuts over the top to serve.

Substitutions

Polenta: wholewheat pasta

Honey: maple syrup

Parmesan: 3 tbsp nutritional yeast or 1 tbsp white miso paste

MUSHROOMS AL PASTOR WITH FENNEL SLAW

Serves 4

Prep time: 10 minutes, plus marinating
Cook time: 30 minutes

These are really delicious, meaty mushrooms in a richly flavoured marinade, combined with a fresh, punchy and tangy slaw. Paired with creamy avocado and fiery green jalapeños, this is a dish the whole family will love. To make this gluten free, simply use whole corn tortillas and tamari.

1kg mixed mushrooms (shiitake and oyster work best), torn or sliced into thin strips

For the marinade

3 tbsp olive oil

2 tbsp tamari or **soy sauce**

1 tbsp tomato purée

2 tsp maple syrup or **molasses**

2 tsp chipotle paste

Juice of 1 lime

3 garlic cloves, crushed

2 tsp ground cumin

For the slaw

1 white onion, thinly sliced

½ white cabbage (400g), shredded

1 large fennel bulb (340g), shredded

1–2 fresh green jalapeños or **green chillies**, thinly sliced

Finely grated zest of 1 lime and **juice of 2 limes**

1 tbsp extra virgin olive oil

2 tsp dried oregano

Pinch each of salt and sugar

To serve

8 small corn tortillas, warmed

150g baby gem lettuce, shredded

1–2 avocados, sliced

Preheat the oven to 200°C fan.

Tip the marinade ingredients, with some freshly ground black pepper, into a large roasting tin and stir together. Roughly tear the mushrooms into the roasting tin, then give everything a really good mix, making sure the mushrooms are evenly coated in the marinade. Roast for 30 minutes, stirring halfway through the cooking time.

Meanwhile, to make the slaw, combine all the ingredients in a large bowl and massage everything with your hands for 5 minutes until the vegetables start to soften. Set aside to marinate for 20 minutes.

Serve the mushrooms with the slaw, warm corn tortillas, shredded lettuce and diced avocado.

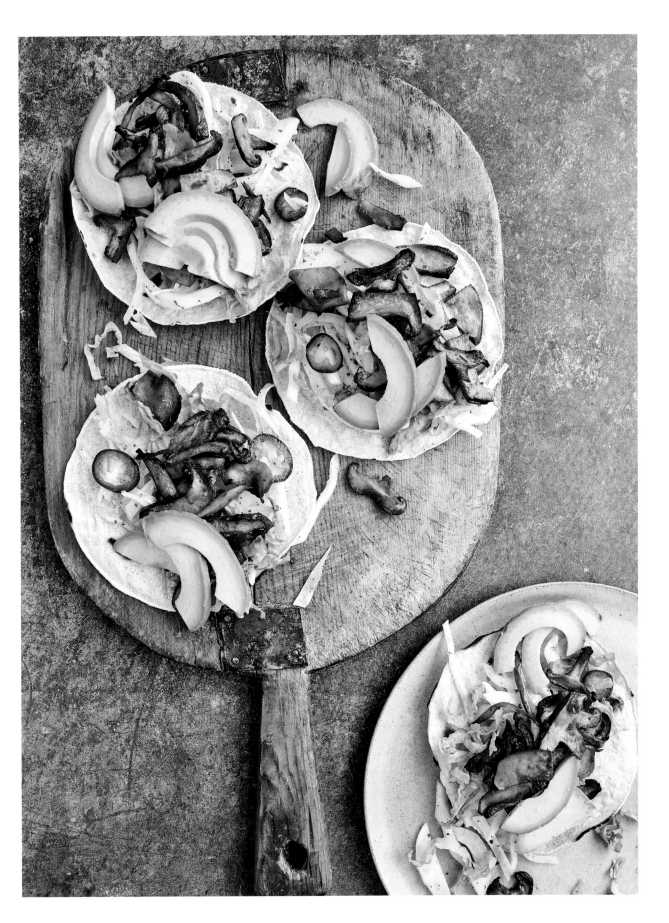

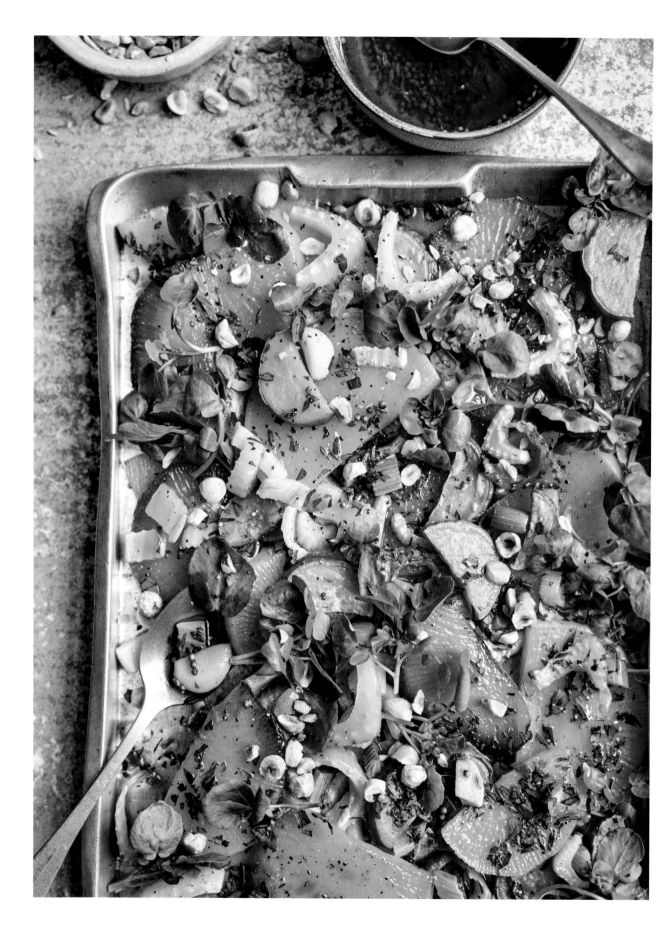

ROAST ROOT VEGETABLES WITH CONFIT GARLIC

Serves 3 to 4 as a side

Prep time: 20 minutes
Cook time: 40 minutes

This super-simple roast vegetable dish is made effortlessly elegant with confit garlic, hints of aromatic coriander and fennel and the subtle heat of paprika. The garlic-infused oil is so useful to keep for other dishes and will elevate the flavour of your cooking.

1 swede (600g), peeled, halved and sliced 5mm thick

3 tbsp extra virgin olive oil

2 small fennel bulbs (400g), sliced 1cm thick

1 sweet potato (240g), scrubbed and unpeeled, halved and sliced 1cm thick

1 tbsp red wine vinegar

50g hazelnuts, toasted and chopped

20g parsley, finely chopped

100g watercress, roughly chopped

For the confit garlic

10 garlic cloves, peeled

2 tsp coriander seeds

2 tsp fennel seeds

200–250ml extra virgin olive oil

½ tsp smoked paprika

Note
Keep any oil left over from making the confit garlic for use in future recipes – it's perfect for drizzling over salads and blanched vegetables. Leave it to cool completely then pour into an airtight container and store in the fridge.

Preheat the oven to 200°C fan.

Tip the swede into a large roasting tin. Drizzle with half the oil and season. Roast for 35 to 40 minutes until soft and caramelised, giving everything a stir halfway through the cooking time.

Put the fennel and sweet potato into another roasting tin with the remaining oil and seasoning. Put into the oven 10 minutes after the swede, so they roast for 25 to 30 minutes and are ready at the same time.

Meanwhile, tip the garlic cloves into a small saucepan, add the coriander and fennel seeds and pour over the oil; the garlic should be completely covered so top up with more oil if needed.

Bring to a gentle simmer then turn the heat down as low as possible and cook for 15 minutes until the garlic is completely soft. Remove from the heat, stir in the smoked paprika and season with salt and pepper. Set aside to cool. (If the garlic starts to brown, take off the heat earlier; you want it to simmer not burn.)

Combine the roasted swede, fennel and sweet potato in one platter. Drain the garlic, reserving the oil, then add the cloves to the roast vegetables along with the vinegar, hazelnuts and parsley. Add 1 or 2 tablespoons of the reserved garlic oil and toss together. Season to taste and serve.

SATAY SQUASH WITH CRISPY CAULIFLOWER

Serves 3 to 4

Prep time: 20 minutes
Cook time: 35 minutes

An easy traybake with a delicious, deeply rich sauce that is super-easy to make and has all the flavours you want in an indulgent satay dressing. I make this once a week; it's filling, and any leftovers heat really well, plus it packs in a huge amount of plant diversity per portion.

2 tbsp coconut oil

1 **small butternut squash**, peeled, deseeded and cut into 2cm cubes (450g prepped weight)

2 tsp **tamari** or **soy sauce**

30g **fresh ginger**, roughly sliced

3 **garlic cloves**, roughly chopped

1 tsp **Sichuan peppercorns**

½ tsp **ground turmeric**

1 tsp **chilli flakes**

1 **leek** (180g), sliced into 2cm rounds

½ **cauliflower** (300g), separated into small florets and leaves

200g **cooked edamame beans** (frozen or from a packet)

For the satay sauce

60g **crunchy peanut butter**

60g **coconut cream**

500ml **boiling water**

1 tbsp **tamari** or **soy sauce**

Juice of 1 lime

To serve

200g **steamed short-grain brown rice**

Lime wedges

50g **spring onions**, sliced on an angle

Preheat the oven to 200°C fan. Place a large roasting tin in the oven for a few minutes to warm.

Put the coconut oil into the roasting tin to melt. Tip in the squash and add the tamari or soy sauce, ginger, garlic, Sichuan peppercorns, turmeric, chilli flakes and coconut oil, then toss well to coat. Roast for 10 minutes, stirring occasionally.

Remove the roasting tin from the oven and add the leek, cauliflower and edamame, basting them in the tray juices.

Return to the oven for a further 20 to 25 minutes until the vegetables are cooked and crispy.

Meanwhile, whisk the satay sauce ingredients together in a small bowl.

Remove the roasting tin from the oven and mix half the satay sauce through the cooked vegetables.

Serve the veggies with the steamed brown rice, lime wedges, spring onions and the remaining satay sauce on the side.

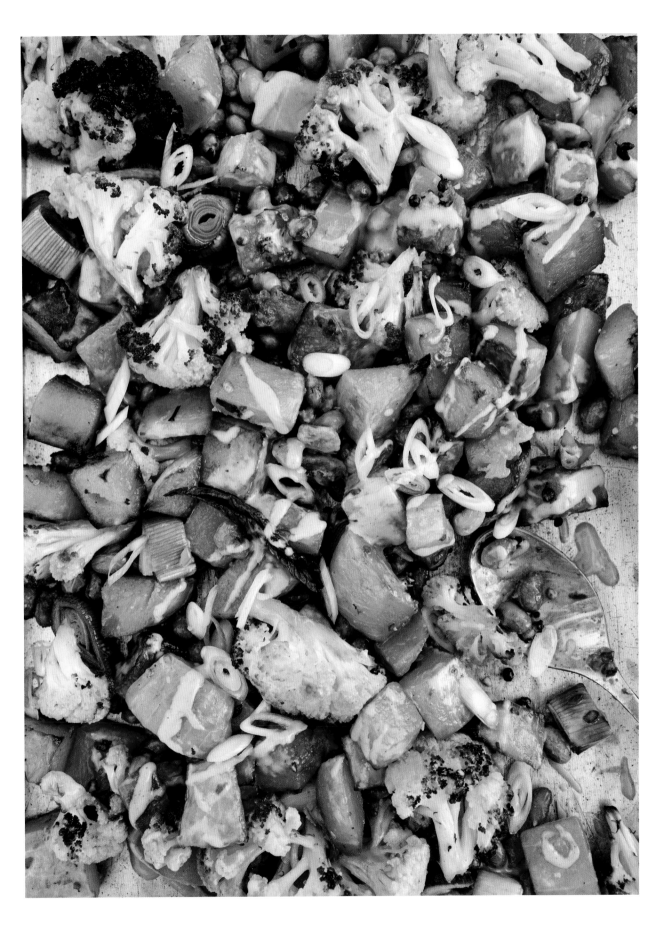

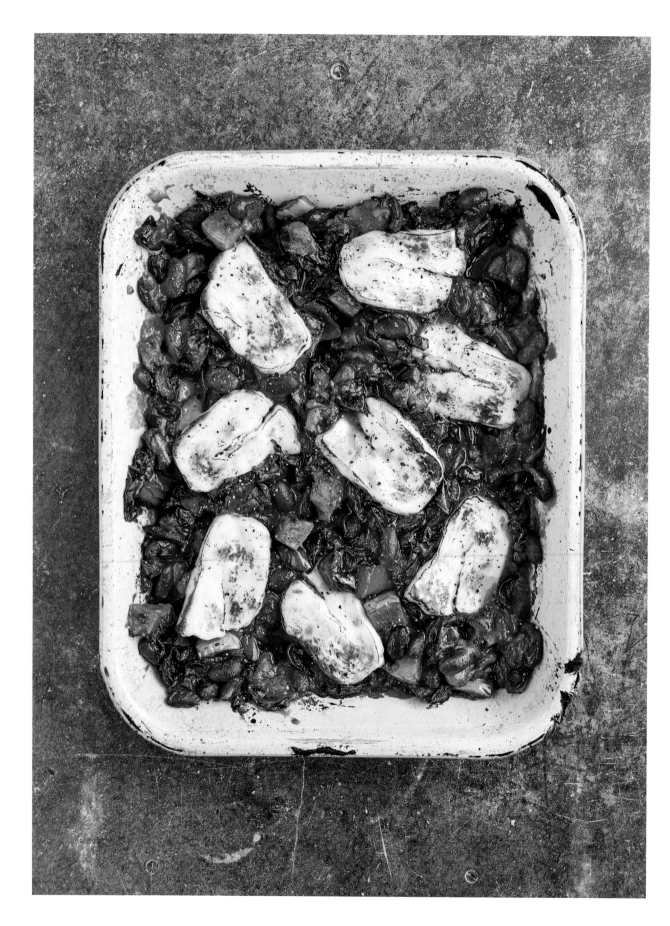

SPICY HALLOUMI BAKE

Prep time: 15 minutes
Cook time: 40 minutes

This is spicy, wholesome, warm and inviting, all in a dish. The beautiful spices of ras el hanout work super-well in this simple traybake and you can easily substitute different vegetables for the squash and greens. A moreish dish packed with flavour that everyone will enjoy.

½ **butternut squash** (300g), scrubbed and unpeeled, deseeded and cut into 2cm cubes

1 **courgette** (250g), cut into 2cm cubes

1 **red pepper** (200g), deseeded and roughly chopped

2 tsp **cumin seeds**

3 tsp **ras el hanout** or **baharat spice mix**

1 tsp **chilli powder**

3 tbsp **olive oil**, plus an extra 1 tbsp to drizzle

150g **spinach**, finely chopped

350ml **passata**

1 x 400g can **kidney beans**, drained and rinsed

200g **halloumi**, sliced 1cm thick

Substitutions

Kale: spinach, Swiss chard or spring greens

Kidney beans: borlotti beans or cannellini beans

Preheat the oven to 200°C fan.

Put the squash, courgette, red pepper and the spices into a large roasting tin. Pour over the 3 tablespoons oil and season, then toss well to coat. Roast for 25 minutes, turning the vegetables halfway through the cooking time.

Remove the roasting tin from the oven and increase the temperature to 220°C fan. Scrape up any crusty bits from the bottom of the roasting tin for extra flavour, then fold in the spinach. Tip in the passata and kidney beans and combine with the rest of the ingredients.

Layer the halloumi on top, drizzle with the extra tablespoon oil and return to the oven for a further 15 minutes until the halloumi is melted and charred in areas.

STICKY BAKED BEANS & VEGETARIAN SAUSAGES

Serves 2

Prep time: 10 minutes
Cook time: 35 minutes

Big, bold flavours are packed into this dish that I love to make on the weekend, but it also serves as a great midweek, no-fuss meal that's packed with four portions of vegetables per serving and deep, indulgent, rich flavours. The soy sauce and honey give a delicious sticky sweet flavour and starting off the dish in the pan gives the spices a chance to infuse into the onions and garlic, as well as making them naturally sweeter.

2 tbsp olive oil, plus an extra drizzle for the sausages

200g red onion, sliced

3 garlic cloves, thinly sliced

200g cavolo nero, leaves stripped and roughly chopped

1 tsp ground cinnamon

1 tsp Cajun or **Creole spice mix**

1 tsp chilli flakes

1 tsp dried thyme

1 tbsp balsamic vinegar or **red wine vinegar**

2 tbsp tomato purée

1 tbsp tamari or **soy sauce**

1 tbsp maple syrup or **honey**

1 x 400g can chopped tomatoes

1 x 400g can haricot beans, drained and rinsed

4 good-quality vegetarian/vegan sausages

10g parsley, finely chopped

Preheat the oven to 200°C fan.

Heat the oil in a large, shallow flameproof casserole over a medium heat and sauté the onion for 5 minutes. Add the garlic, greens and some seasoning, and toss with the onions for a further 2 to 3 minutes, to gently cook the greens.

Add the spices and thyme cook for a minute before adding the vinegar, tomato purée, tamari or soy sauce, honey or maple syrup, tomatoes and beans. Stir through the ingredients and bring to a simmer for 2 to 3 minutes, adding a splash of water (about 50ml) to loosen the mixture.

Lay the sausages on top, drizzle over a little more oil and season. Roast in the oven for 25 minutes, giving everything a quick stir halfway through the cooking time, until the tomatoes begin to brown at the edges and the sausages are golden and cooked in the sauce.

Scatter over the parsley to serve.

Substitutions

Vegetarian sausages: good-quality, minimally processed regular sausages

Cavolo nero: Spring greens, hispi cabbage or curly kale

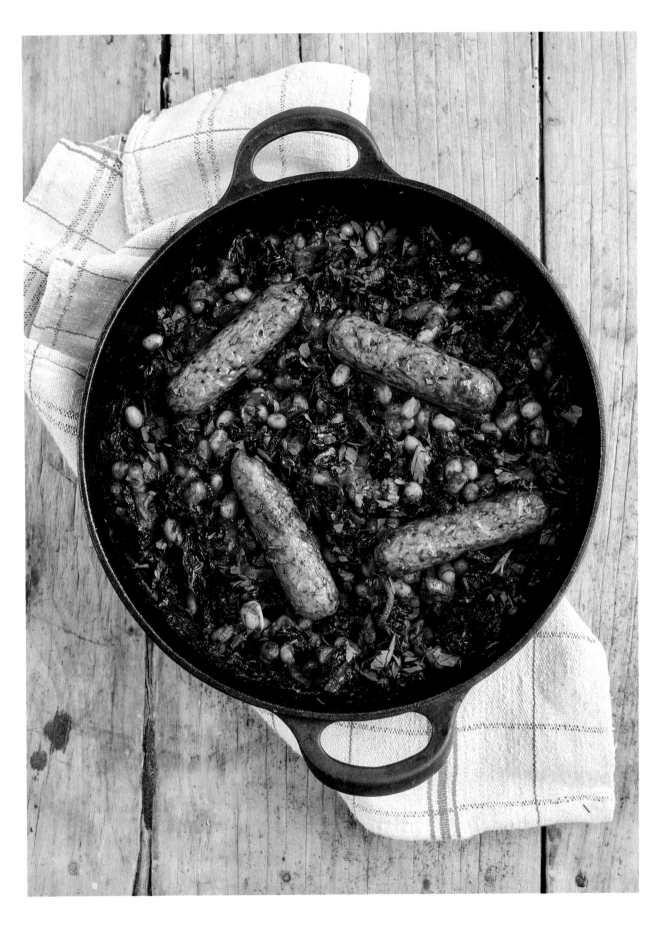

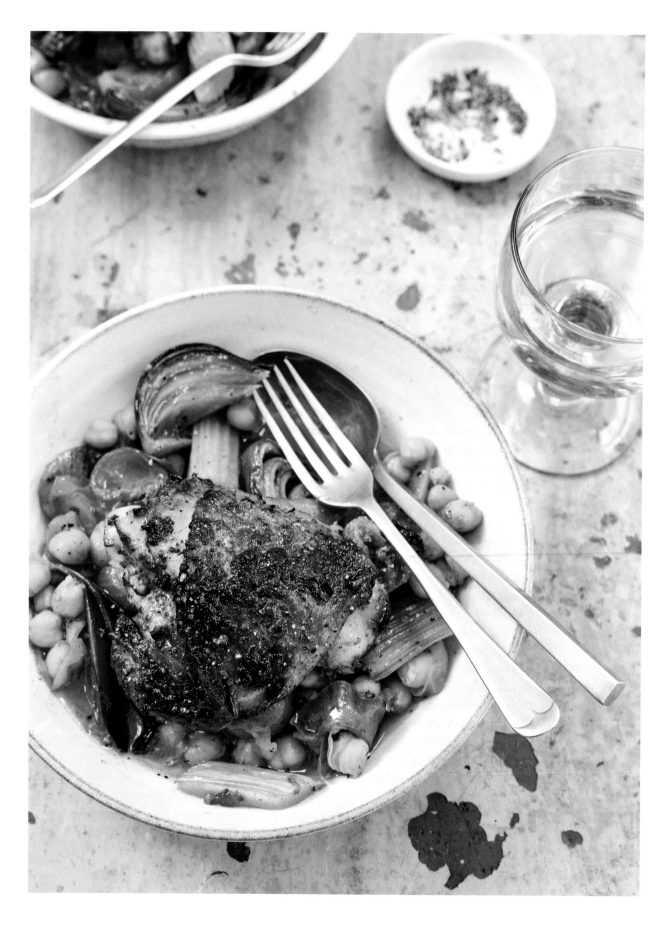

CRISPY SUMAC CHICKEN

Serves 2 to 3

Prep time: 15 minutes, plus marinating
Cook time: 50 minutes

In my household, we see this as a bit of a luxury dish. I'm mostly plant-based, but sometimes you just crave the delicious flavour of roasted chicken with the amalgamation of molasses, earthy warming spices and tangy sumac. The vegetables cook down into a stew, with the flavours from the marinade adding all the elements you need to make this wonderful dish.

2 bone-in, skin-on chicken thighs (400g)

200g red onion, cut into wedges

200g celery, cut into thick chunks

300g baby tomatoes, halved

Drizzle of olive oil

1x 400g can chickpeas, drained and rinsed

For the marinade

2 tbsp olive oil

2 tsp sumac

1 tsp coriander seeds, freshly ground

1 tsp cumin seeds, freshly ground

1 tsp cinnamon

½ tsp chilli flakes

3 garlic cloves, grated

1 tbsp red wine vinegar

1 tbsp date molasses or **pomegranate molasses**

Preheat the oven to 200°C fan.

Mix the marinade ingredients together in a bowl with salt and pepper to taste. Thoroughly coat the chicken thighs in the marinade and leave for at least 10 minutes (but the longer you leave the chicken in the marinade, the better.)

Put the onion, celery and tomatoes into large a roasting tin with the oil and a pinch each of salt and pepper. Lay the marinated chicken on top and stir any remaining marinade through the vegetables. Roast in the oven for 30 minutes.

Remove the roasting tin from the oven and add the chickpeas, stirring them through the vegetables. Return to the oven for a further 20 minutes until the chicken skin is deeply coloured and crispy on top.

Serve the stewed chickpeas in bowls with the chicken on top.

HARISSA & ZA'ATAR SEAFOOD TRAYBAKE

Serves 2

Prep time: 20 minutes
Cook time: 30 minutes

A simple traybake I make often with different seasonal ingredients or depending on what I have to hand in my groceries. It's herby, sweet, spicy and wholesome, with a fantastic mix of fibre-rich vegetables.

1 onion (180g), sliced

1 small fennel bulb (200g), sliced

1 lemon, sliced

2 tbsp extra virgin olive oil

300g mixed skinless fish
(salmon, monkfish, haddock), cut into 3cm cubes

1 tbsp harissa paste

For the freekeh

100g freekeh

1 tbsp extra virgin olive oil

250ml boiling water

100g spinach, roughly chopped

200g chickpeas, from a jar, drained and rinsed

Juice of ½ lemon

2 tsp za'atar, plus extra to serve

To serve

Small bunch of parsley, finely chopped

Lemon wedges

Substitution

Freekah: short-grain brown rice

Preheat the oven to 180°C fan. Place a large roasting tin in the oven for a few minutes to warm.

Tip the onion, fennel and lemon into the roasting tin. Drizzle with the oil, season and toss well to coat. Roast for 20 minutes, giving everything a stir halfway through the cooking time.

Toss the cubed fish in the harissa paste, making sure everything is evenly coated, then arrange in an even layer over the vegetables. Return to the oven for a further 8 to 10 minutes until the fish flakes easily when pressed.

Meanwhile, add the freekeh to a dry saucepan over a medium heat and toast the grains lightly for a minute before adding the olive oil and boiling water.

Simmer for 25 minutes (or according to the packet instructions), then stir through the spinach for 1 minute until wilted. Add the chickpeas, lemon juice, za'atar, and season with salt and pepper.

Spoon the freekeh into bowls and top with the vegetables and fish. Scatter over the parsley and a little more za'atar. Serve with lemon wedges.

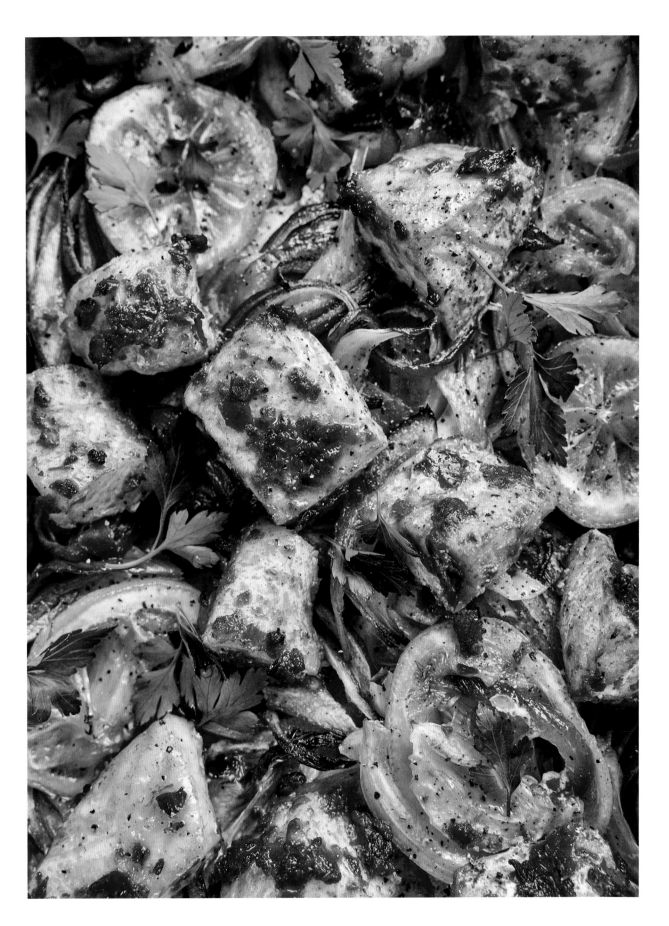

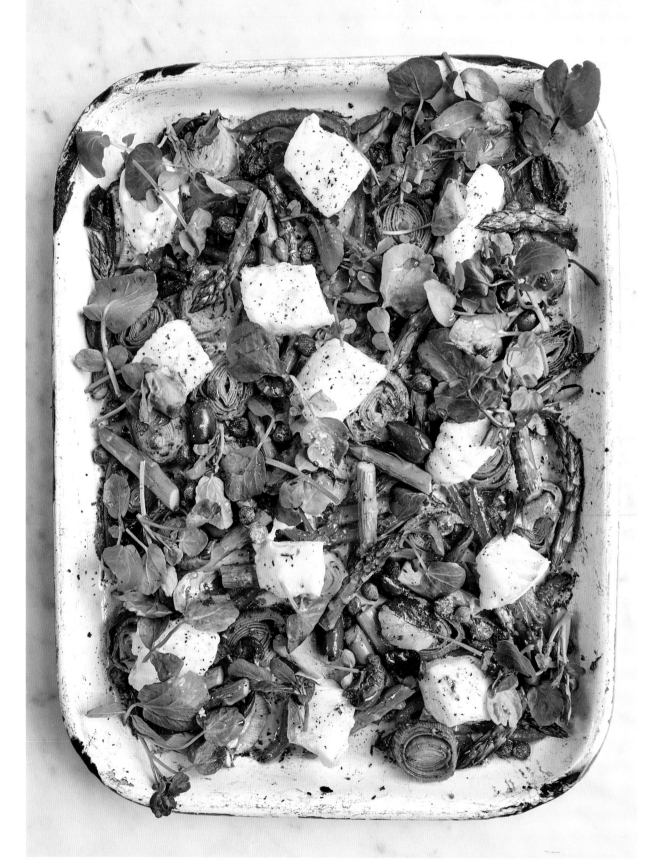

MEDITERRANEAN FISH TRAYBAKE

Serves 2 generously

Prep time: 15 minutes
Cook time: 30 minutes

This simple traybake has a gorgeous mix of saltiness from the capers and olives, sweetness from the roasted leek and pepper, with a hint of spice from the chilli. The herbs round it off nicely and you will love the ease of this dish.

1 leek (160g), sliced 1cm thick

1 red pepper (160g), deseeded and thinly sliced

3 garlic cloves, grated

2 sprigs of rosemary, leaves chopped

1 red chilli, thinly sliced

2 tsp dried oregano

2 tbsp extra virgin olive oil

160g asparagus spears, roughly cut into 3cm lengths

250g skinless, firm white fish, such as cod, monkfish or sea bass, cut into 3cm cubes

50g pitted Kalamata olives, roughly torn

2 tbsp capers

100g watercress, roughly torn

Preheat the oven to 180°C fan. Place a large roasting tin in the oven for a few minutes to warm.

Tip the leek, pepper, garlic, rosemary, chilli and oregano into the roasting tin. Drizzle with the oil and season, then toss well to coat. Roast for 10 minutes.

Add the asparagus, giving everything a stir, and cook for a further 10 minutes.

Remove the roasting tin from the oven and stir the fish, olives and capers through the vegetables. Return to the oven for a further 6 to 8 minutes until the fish flakes easily when pressed.

Scatter over the chopped watercress and serve.

CAULIFLOWER, FENNEL & SALMON TRAYBAKE

Serves 2

Prep time: 20 minutes
Cook time: 40 minutes

A light, fresh and tangy meal with a sharp citrus and fennel seed flavour that cuts through the oily salmon. A perfect midweek meal packed with health-promoting ingredients, including anti-inflammatory omega-3 fats.

½ **cauliflower** (300g), separated into small florets and leaves

1 **medium fennel bulb** (250g), thinly sliced, fronds reserved

4 **garlic cloves**, unpeeled

2 **tbsp olive oil**

200g **fine green beans**

1 **lemon**, ½ sliced and the remaining ½ quartered into wedges, to serve

1 **tsp nigella seeds**

1 **tsp fennel seeds**, crushed

2 x 150g **salmon fillets**, skin scored

8 **cornichons** or **mini gherkins**, finely chopped

Small bunch of tarragon, leaves chopped

Substitutions

Cornichons: 1 tbsp capers

Preheat the oven to 180°C fan. Place a large roasting tin in the oven for a few minutes to warm.

Tip the cauliflower, fennel and garlic into the tin. Drizzle with the olive oil, season with salt and pepper, then toss well to coat. Roast for 10 minutes, stirring occasionally.

Stir in the green beans, lemon slices, nigella and fennel seeds, and roast for a further 15 minutes.

Remove the roasting tin from the oven and increase the temperature to 200°C fan. Lay the salmon fillets on top of the vegetables, skin-side up, add a drizzle of oil and season well.

Return the roasting tin to the oven for a further 12 to 15 minutes until the salmon is just cooked through.

Transfer the salmon to a plate and keep warm. Slip the garlic cloves from their skins and stir through the roasted vegetables, along with the cornichons and tarragon.

Pile the roasted vegetables onto plates and lay the salmon on top. Scatter over the reserved fennel fronds and serve with the lemon wedges.

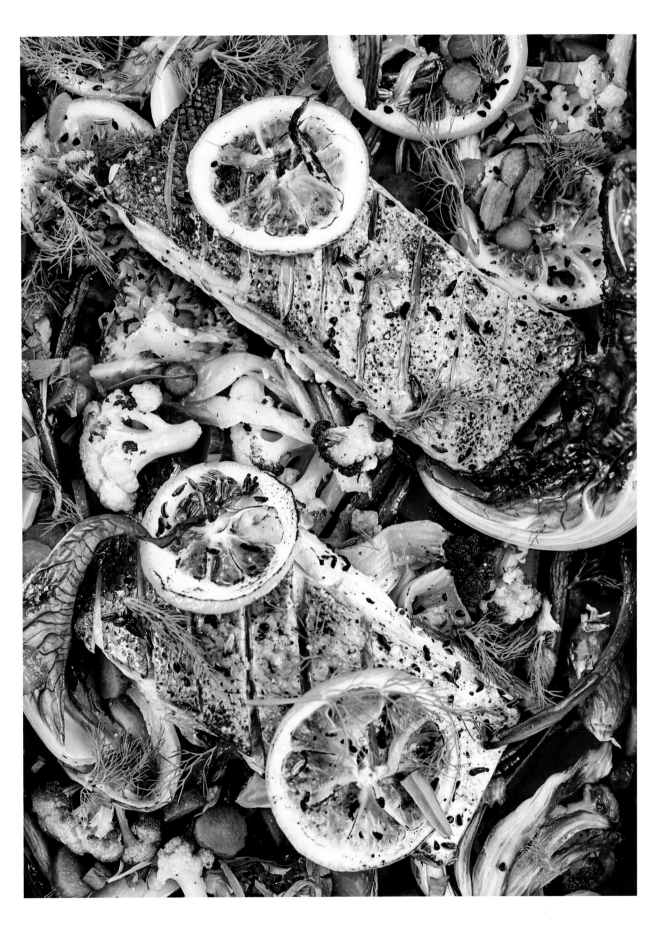

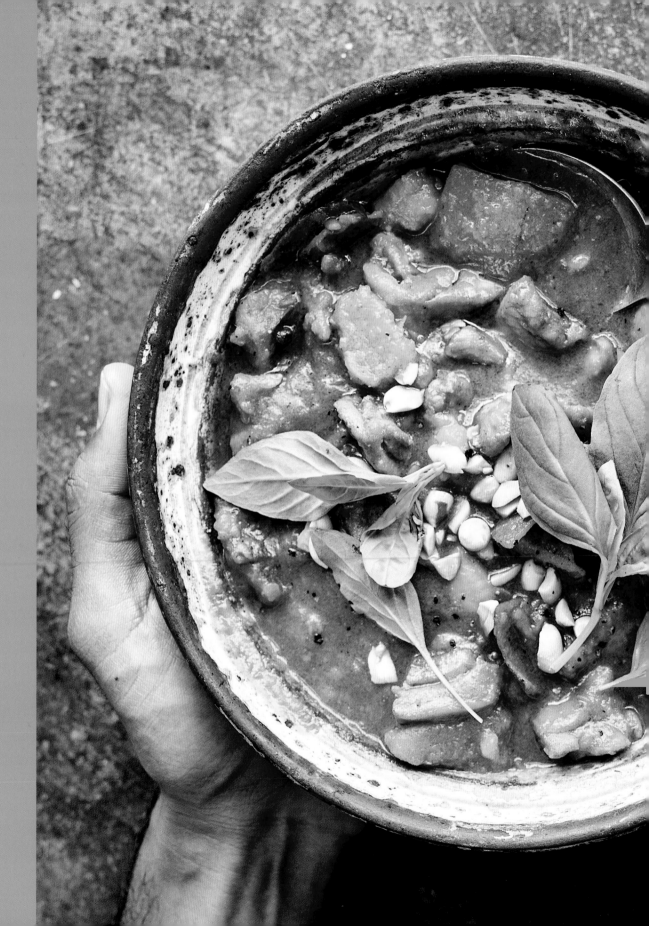

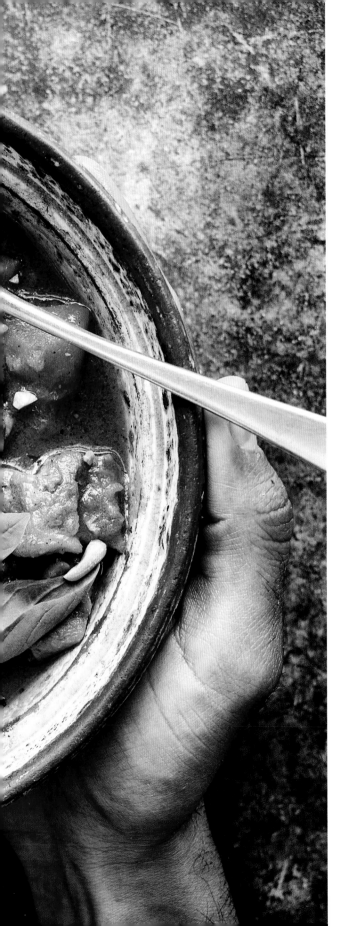

CURRIES

AUBERGINE, PEA & TAMARIND CURRY

Serves 4

Prep time: 20 minutes
Cook time: 30 minutes

I love this sweet, tangy curry packed with warming masala spices and plenty of vegetables. It's my go-to recipe for a midweek meal with no fuss. Recipe testers described this curry as an unexpectedly delicious and flavourful meal with a meaty texture, luscious thick sauce and the citrus tang of the tamarind contrasting beautifully with the smooth almond butter. This will become your new favourite curry!

2–3 aubergines (500g), cut into 2cm thick chunks

2 tbsp coconut oil, melted

2 tsp each cumin seeds, fennel seeds and **black mustard seeds**

1 cinnamon stick

12 curry leaves (optional)

2 tsp garam masala

4 garlic cloves, chopped

25g fresh ginger, grated

400g tomatoes, chopped

1–2 small green chillies, sliced

3 tbsp tamarind paste

3 tbsp smooth almond butter

200ml boiling water

400g frozen peas, thawed

To serve

20g coriander, chopped

Plain chapatti or **roti** (see page 203 for homemade)

Preheat the oven to 200°C fan.

Put the aubergine in a large roasting tin (or split it between two tins) with 1 tablespoon of the coconut oil and a pinch of salt, then toss to coat in the oil. Roast in the oven for 20 minutes, turning halfway through the cooking time, until golden and soft.

Meanwhile, heat the remaining oil in a heavy-based pan over a medium heat, add the whole spices and curry leaves, if using, and fry for 1 to 2 minutes. Add the garam masala, garlic and ginger and fry for a further 2 to 3 minutes. Stir in the tomatoes and chillies and let everything bubble up and simmer for 5 minutes, or until the tomatoes start to break down.

Stir in the tamarind, almond butter and boiling water and bring to a simmer. Add the roasted aubergine pieces to the pan, cover with a lid and cook gently for a further 10 minutes. Add the peas for the last 5 minutes of cooking time.

Remove from the heat and season to taste. To serve, spoon the curry into bowls, scatter over the chopped coriander and serve with chapatti or roti.

Note

If you haven't got all the spices, don't worry. The most important spice is the garam masala with all the rich polyphenols you find in cinnamon, cumin and chilli.

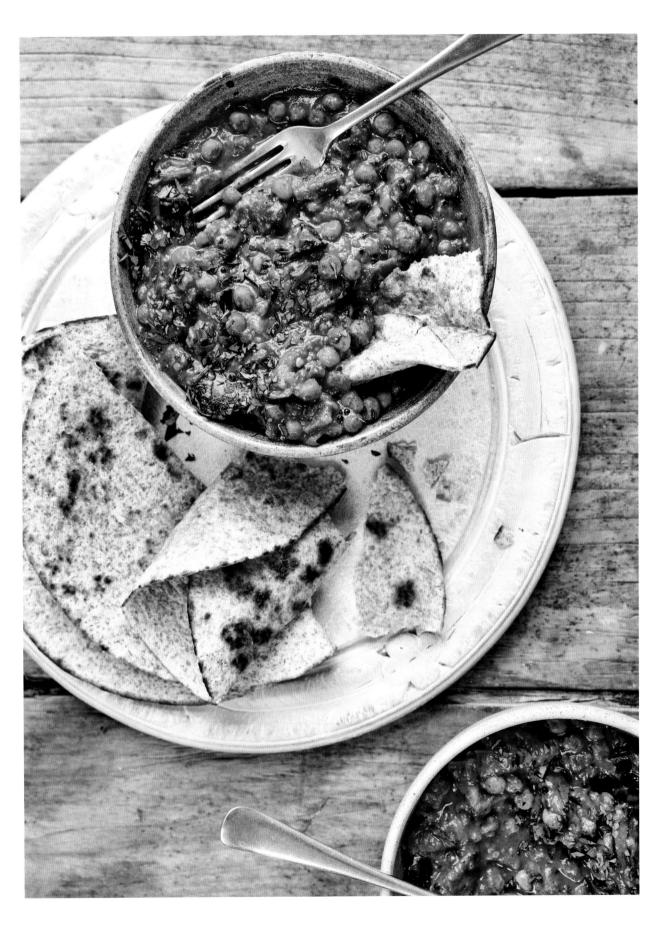

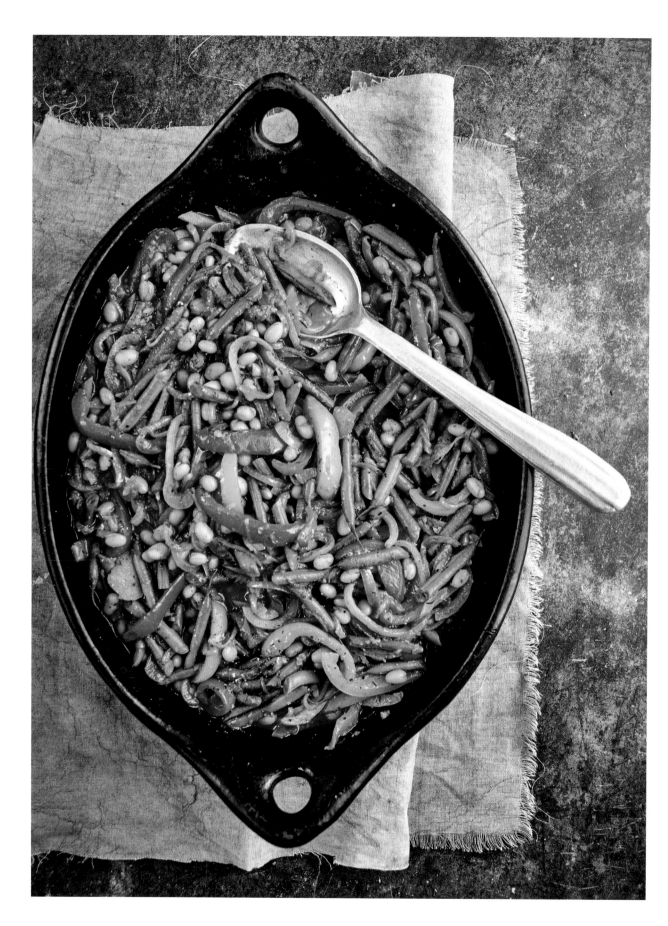

CHAKALAKA CURRIED VEGGIE BEANS

Serves 4

Prep time: 15 minutes
Cook time: 25 minutes

With delicate curry spices and crunchy green beans, this appetising bean stew is super-easy to put together for a midweek meal or batch cook for the freezer. The ginger and cayenne pepper combine to give the curry a subtle heat, while the quantity of fibre-rich ingredients it contains will keep your gut microbes thriving.

3 tbsp olive oil

500g mixed peppers, deseeded and sliced

2 onions (360g), thinly sliced

4 garlic cloves, grated

40g fresh ginger, grated

30g tomato purée

1 tbsp curry powder

2 tsp dried thyme

2 tsp smoked paprika

1 tsp cayenne pepper or chilli powder

2 x 400g cans haricot beans, drained and rinsed

1 vegetable stock cube

250ml hot water

200g green beans, roughly chopped

Heat the oil in a deep frying pan over a medium heat. Add the sliced peppers and onions and fry for 6 to 7 minutes, stirring regularly, until softened. Add the garlic, ginger, tomato purée and spices, fry for 2 minutes then tip in the haricot beans.

Crumble in the stock cube and pour over the hot water. Bring to a simmer then cover with a lid and cook for 10 minutes.

Stir in the green beans, cover and cook for a further 5 minutes. Remove from the heat, season to taste and then serve.

Substitutions

Haricot beans: mixed beans or chickpeas

Green beans: frozen beans (thawed)

KALA CHANA

Prep time: 15 minutes
Cook time: 30 minutes

Tasty, homely and authentic are the words that come to mind when I describe this flavour-packed simple dish. Kala chana are firmer and nuttier than regular chickpeas and have a higher fibre content, but you can easily use regular chickpeas in this recipe. Blending some of the mixture adds a rich creamy texture without the traditional use of chunks of butter or ghee! Serve this curry with brown rice or flatbreads.

2 tbsp **avocado oil** or **coconut oil**

2 **small red onions** (300g), diced

6 **cardamom pods**, bruised

1 **cinnamon stick**

40g **fresh ginger**, grated

3 **garlic cloves**, grated

2 tsp **ground coriander**

2 tsp **ground cumin**

1–2 tsp **chilli powder**

2 x 400g cans **kala chana (black chickpeas)**, drained and rinsed

500ml **vegetable stock**

200g **spinach**, roughly chopped

To serve

2 tbsp **natural yoghurt**

2 tsp **garam masala**

Heat the oil in a large saucepan over a medium heat, add the onions, cardamom pods and cinnamon stick with some seasoning and sauté for 6 to 7 minutes until soft. Add the grated ginger, garlic, ground coriander, cumin and chilli powder, and fry for 1 minute.

Add the kala chana and stock to the pan and bring to a simmer, then cover with a lid and cook for 15 minutes.

Transfer a ladleful of the chana and cooking liquid to a jug. Using a stick blender, blitz the chana until smooth. Pour the blended chana back into the pan, stir in the spinach leaves and let them cook for 2 to 3 minutes until wilted. Remove the pan from the heat and season to taste.

To serve, spoon the curry into bowls and then dot the yoghurt on top and add a dusting of garam masala.

Substitutions

Kala chana: regular chickpeas, black beans or navy beans

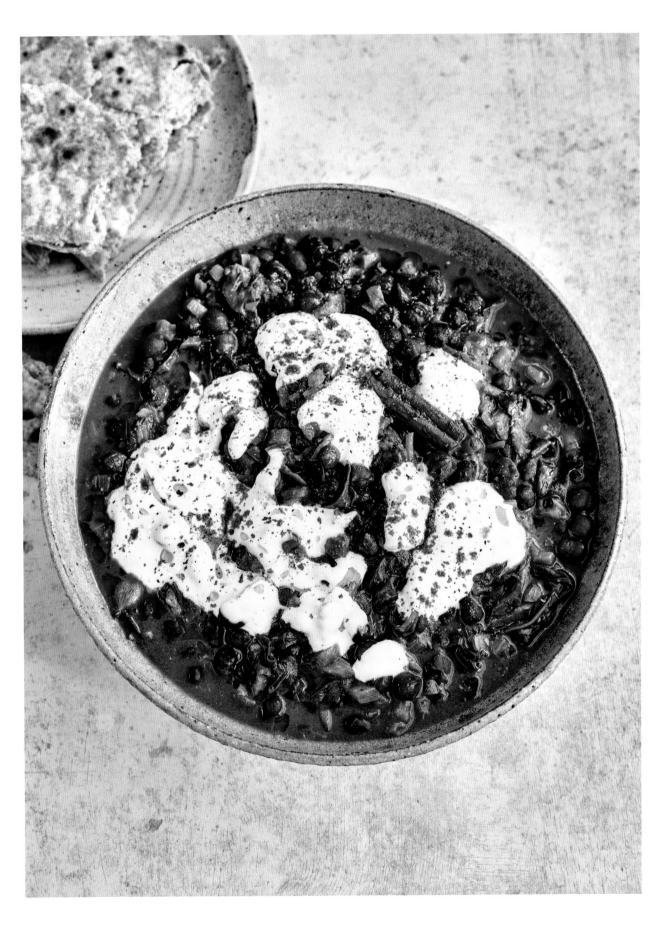

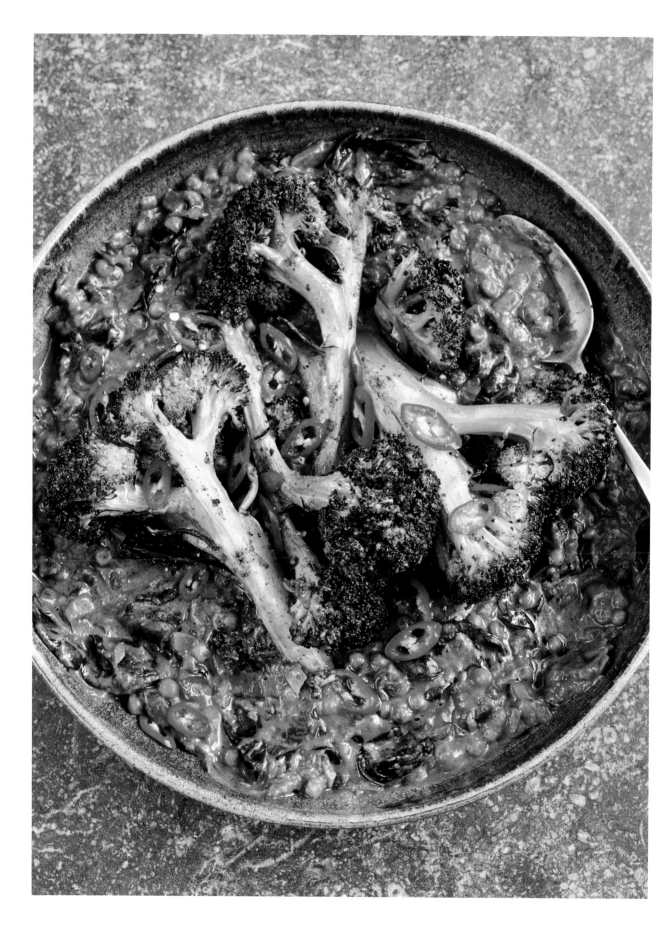

GINGER PEANUT CURRY WITH ROASTED BROCCOLI

Serves 2

Prep time: 10 minutes
Cook time: 40 minutes

At least once a week I eat this gingery, peanutty curry with sweet roasted tomatoes, fresh greens and beautifully crisp broccoli on top. This meal has so much flavour, delicious spices and contrasting textures, plus it contains more than five portions of vegetables per serving.

4 tbsp olive oil, plus extra to drizzle

3 garlic cloves, grated

3 tsp garam masala

1 small head broccoli (about 350g), quartered

300g baby tomatoes, halved

1 large red onion (about 160g), diced

30g fresh ginger, grated

1 tsp cumin seeds, freshly ground

½ tsp ground cinnamon

½ tsp ground turmeric

1 tsp sweet paprika

1 vegetable stock cube

500ml hot water

2 tbsp peanut butter (with no added oil, salt or sugar)

100g peas (fresh or frozen, thawed)

100g spinach

1 red chilli, finely sliced on an angle, to garnish

Preheat the oven to 200°C fan.

In a roasting tin, whisk together 2 tablespoons of the olive oil, the grated garlic and garam masala. Add the broccoli pieces to the tin and toss to coat in the oil mixture. Pop the tomatoes in the tin and then lay the broccoli on top. Season well and drizzle over a little more olive oil then roast in the oven for 30 to 35 minutes, checking halfway through the cooking time and turning the broccoli as needed.

When the broccoli is halfway through roasting, warm the remaining oil in a large saucepan over a medium heat. Add the onion and sauté for 5 minutes. Add the grated ginger and ground spices, then cook for a further 2 to 3 minutes until the onion is infused with their flavours.

Add the stock cube, hot water and peanut butter to the pan with the onion and bring to a gentle simmer. Setting the roasted broccoli aside, scrape the tomatoes out of the tin into the pan with the simmering curry and stir through (if the curry is too thick for your liking, add more hot water).

Add the peas to the curry and let them warm through, then throw in the spinach and let it gently wilt in the heat for 1 minute. Remove the pan from the heat. To serve, spoon the curry into bowls, then top each bowl with the roasted broccoli and sliced red chilli.

GOAN-STYLE SPICED BLACK BEAN CURRY

Serves 4

Prep time: 15 minutes
Cook time: 30 minutes

The ginger, cardamom and curry leaf flavours with a kick of spice and coconut is a beautiful combination for this sauce and pairs well with the sweet shallot. Cooking the greens right at the end preserves their vibrancy, vitamin C and fresh flavour.

2 tbsp coconut oil

2 shallots (120g), thinly sliced

4 garlic cloves, grated

40g fresh ginger, grated

3 tsp cumin seeds

2 tsp black mustard seeds

2 dried Kashmiri chillies, stalks and seeds removed, crumbled

4 cardamom pods, bashed

10–12 curry leaves

1 tsp ground turmeric

2 x 400ml cans coconut milk

2 x 400g cans black beans, drained and rinsed

300g kale, stems removed, roughly chopped

300g sugar snap peas, sliced on an angle

Juice of 1 lime

Small bunch of coriander, chopped

1 red chilli, thinly sliced

Lime wedges, to serve

Heat the oil in a saucepan over a medium heat, add the shallots, garlic and ginger and sauté for 5 minutes until soft. Add the cumin seeds, mustard seeds, dried chillies, cardamom pods and curry leaves and fry for 1 minute until fragrant.

Stir in the ground turmeric, coconut milk and black beans. Bring everything to the boil then reduce the heat and simmer gently for 15 minutes.

Stir in the kale, cover with a lid and cook for 5 minutes. Add the sugar snap peas and cook for a further 2 minutes. Remove the pan from the heat, stir in the lime juice and season with a pinch of salt.

To serve, spoon the curry into bowls, scatter over the coriander and sliced chilli and garnish with lime wedges for squeezing.

Substitutions

Dried Kashmiri chillies: 1 tsp chilli powder

Kale: hispi cabbage

Sugar snap peas: green beans or peas

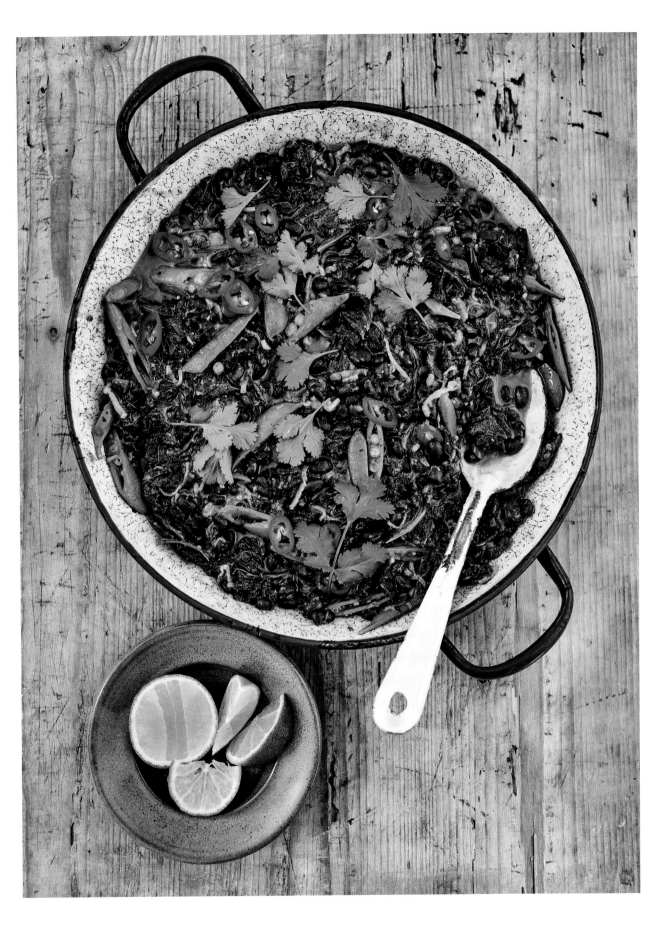

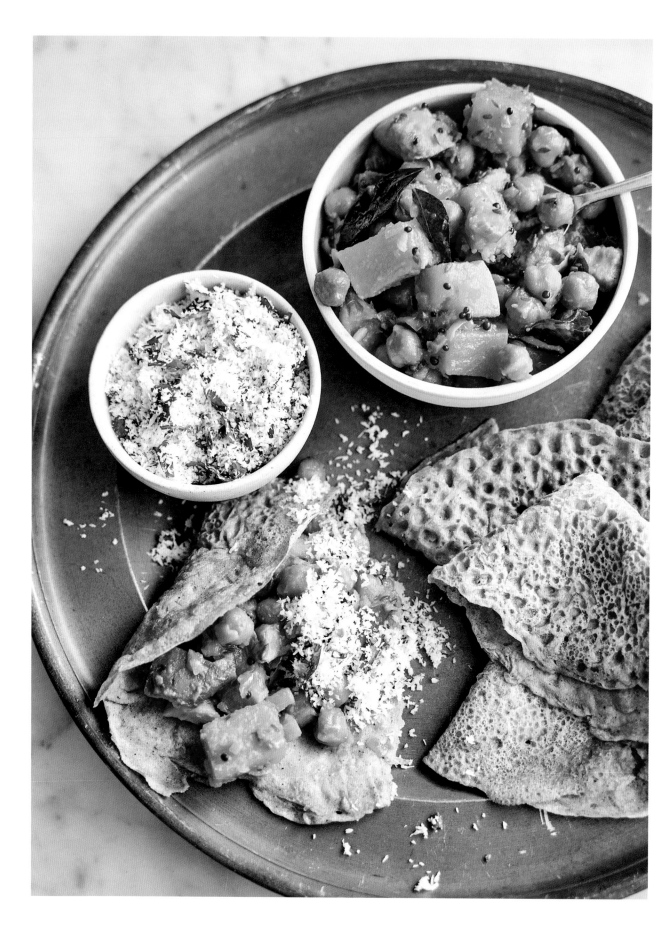

PUMPKIN CURRY WITH PANCAKES & COCONUT CHUTNEY

Serves 3 or 4

Prep time: 20 minutes
Cook time: 40 minutes

If you're not feeling that adventurous, you can skip the buckwheat pancakes because the pumpkin masala curry is gorgeous on its own. The vibrant, zingy coconut chutney is super simple to make and beautifully complements the curry. There is plenty of plant protein in this dish, all harmonised with nutrient-dense spices. If you do omit the pancakes, serve this curry simply with rice.

For the pumpkin masala

2 tsp coconut oil

1 white onion (180g), finely chopped

2 tsp black mustard seeds

2 tsp cumin seeds

12 curry leaves

½ tsp ground turmeric

300g pumpkin or **butternut squash**, skin on, deseeded and cut into 1.5cm cubes

1 large sweet potato (300g), skin on, cut into 1.5cm cubes

1 x 400g can chickpeas, drained and rinsed

50g coconut cream

For the buckwheat pancakes

150g buckwheat flour

1 tsp garam masala

1 tsp salt

2 tbsp coconut oil

For the coconut chutney

50g freshly grated or **desiccated coconut**

Grated zest and **juice of 1 lime**

½ tsp chilli flakes

20g coriander, finely chopped

For the buckwheat pancakes, combine the buckwheat flour, garam masala and salt in a large mixing bowl. Pour in 400ml water and whisk until smooth. Leave to stand while you prepare the pumpkin masala.

For the pumpkin masala, heat the oil in a large sauté pan over medium-high heat. Add the onion and fry gently for 3 to 4 minutes or until softened. Add the mustard seeds, cumin seeds and curry leaves and fry for 1 minute until fragrant. Stir in the ground turmeric and a pinch of salt. Throw in the pumpkin and sweet potato pieces, tossing to coat in the oil and spices. Add the chickpeas and coconut cream, then pour over 200ml water and cover with a lid. Cook gently for 20 minutes or until the vegetables are soft, then set aside and keep warm.

Meanwhile, make the coconut chutney by combining all the ingredients in a small bowl with salt and pepper to taste.

To cook the pancakes, heat a little coconut oil in a non-stick frying pan over a medium heat. Pour in a ladleful of the batter and swirl to coat the base of the pan in a thin, even layer. Cook gently for 2 to 3 minutes on one side or until the edges are lacy, golden and crisp. You should see bubbles appear on the surface of the pancake. Flip the pancake and cook for a further 2 minutes on the other side. Repeat with the remaining batter and oil.

To serve, spoon the pumpkin masala on top of the pancakes and garnish with some of the coconut chutney.

RAJMA MAKHANI

Serves 2 as a main or 4 as a side

Prep time: 15 minutes
Cook time: 35 minutes

For the few ingredients involved in this recipe, the result is a delicious, hearty bean dish with wonderful spiciness and sweetness. The traditional Punjabi dish is made with lashings of cream, but puréeing a little of the beans gives a richness that mimics the original without the heaviness.

2 tbsp **avocado oil** or **olive oil**

1 **onion** (180g), chopped

4 **garlic cloves**, grated

30g fresh ginger, grated

2 small green chillies, thinly sliced, plus extra to serve

3 tsp **garam masala**

300g tomatoes, chopped

2 x 400g cans kidney beans, drained and rinsed

1 **vegetable stock cube**

200ml hot water

To serve

Coconut yoghurt or **natural yoghurt** (optional)

Small bunch of coriander, roughly chopped

Substitutions

Kidney beans: mixed beans, black beans or navy beans

Heat the oil in a wide flameproof casserole over a medium heat. Add the onions, season with salt and pepper and cook gently for 7 to 8 minutes or until softened and beginning to caramelise. Add the garlic, ginger and chillies and fry for 2 to 3 minutes, then stir in the garam masala and fry for a further 1 minute until fragrant.

Add the tomatoes to the pan and cook for 10 minutes or until they start to break down and thicken. Add the kidney beans, stock cube and hot water and bring to a simmer, then cover with a lid and cook gently for 10 minutes.

Transfer a ladleful of the kidney beans and cooking liquid to a jug. Using a stick blender, blitz the beans until smooth. Stir the blended beans back into the pan. Remove the pan from the heat and season with a pinch of salt.

To serve, spoon the curry into individual bowls and then add a swirl of yoghurt, if you like, and scatter over the chopped coriander and chilli.

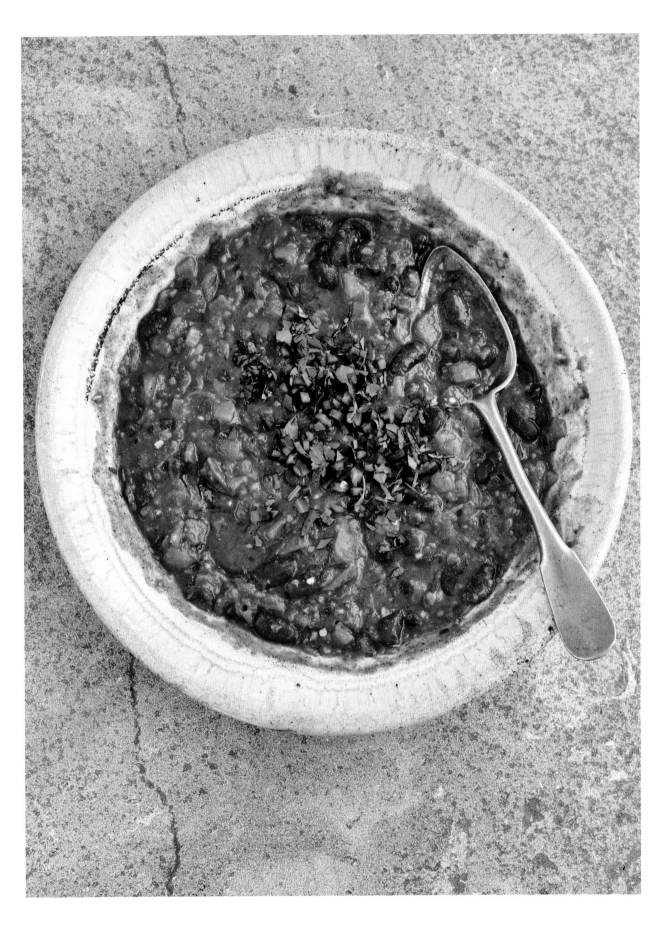

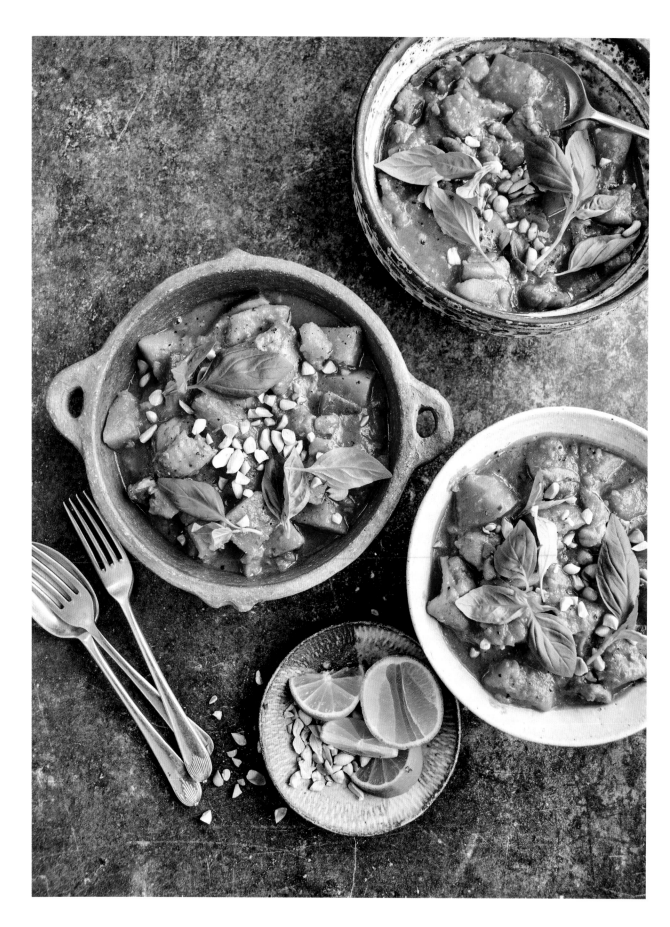

VIETNAMESE-STYLE CHICKEN CURRY

Serves 4

Prep time: 20 minutes, plus marinating
Cook time: 30 minutes

This light chicken curry is perfect when you crave something fragrant. The paste is packed with lemon tang and a balancing touch of sweetness from the sugar. It's easy to turn veggie by replacing the chicken with marinated tempeh and using soy instead of fish sauce.

500g boneless, skinless chicken thighs, cut into bite-sized pieces

1 tbsp Vietnamese curry powder or **mild curry powder**

1 tbsp tamari or **soy sauce**

1 tbsp coconut oil

2 tsp ground turmeric

400g pumpkin or **butternut squash**, peeled and cut into 2cm cubes

400g sweet potato, scrubbed and cut into 2cm cubes

1 x 400ml can coconut milk

2 tsp palm or **coconut sugar**

350g baby leaf spinach, chopped

1–2 tbsp fish sauce

For the curry paste

2 fresh red chillies

4 garlic cloves

3 lemongrass stalks, outer leaves discarded, chopped

30g fresh ginger, chopped

10g coriander, stalks only, leaves reserved to garnish

2 tbsp coconut oil, melted

2 tsp fish sauce (optional)

To serve

Small bunch of Thai basil or **regular basil**, leaves roughly torn

50g unsalted peanuts, chopped

2 limes, cut into wedges

Put the chicken in a large bowl, sprinkle over the curry powder and tamari or soy sauce, then mix thoroughly. Cover and set aside for 20 minutes.

Meanwhile, make the curry paste. Put all the ingredients into a small food processor with 2 tbsp water and blend to a smooth paste.

Heat the oil in a large saucepan over a medium heat, add the curry paste and ground turmeric and fry for 3 to 4 minutes or until fragrant. Add the pumpkin and sweet potato pieces to the pan. (Sometimes pumpkin skin can be pretty tough, which is why I peel it here, but if you use small pumpkins or butternut squash then there's no need to peel them.) Fry for 1 minute, then tip in the coconut milk, 150ml water and sugar. Bring to a simmer and cook for 5 minutes.

Stir in the chicken, then cover with a lid and cook gently for 20 minutes or until the pumpkin is tender but still holding its shape. Stir in the spinach, remove the pan from the heat, then add the fish sauce to taste and check the seasoning.

To serve, spoon the curry into bowls, stir through the coriander leaves and top with the Thai basil leaves, then scatter over the chopped peanuts and garnish with lime wedges on the side.

GARAM MASALA CHICKPEA & CHICKEN CURRY

Serves 4

Prep time: 15 minutes
Cook time: 35 minutes

This dish is creamy, subtly spiced and absolutely gorgeous for a one-pot dish. The flavours intensify with the chicken, and the mild spices and chickpeas give a gentle warmth to the dish that pairs well with the dark greens. The coconut base adds an elegant richness that you will enjoy too.

2 tbsp avocado oil

4 boneless, skinless chicken thighs (350g)

2 onions (300g), chopped

3 garlic cloves, grated

30g fresh ginger, grated

60g ground almonds

2 tsp garam masala

2 tsp sweet paprika

2 tsp black mustard seeds

2 x 400g cans chickpeas, drained and rinsed

1 x 400ml can coconut milk

300g cavolo nero or **spring greens**, stalks removed, leaves roughly chopped

Heat 1 tablespoon of the oil in a wide flameproof casserole over a medium-high heat. Add the chicken thighs and brown for 3 to 4 minutes on each side. Remove from the pan and set aside.

Pour the remaining oil into the pan, add the onions and cook gently for 7 to 8 minutes or until softened and beginning to caramelise. Add the garlic and ginger, fry for 2 to 3 minutes, then stir in the ground almonds, garam masala, paprika and mustard seeds. Season well and fry for 30 seconds until fragrant.

Add the chickpeas to the casserole, then pour in the coconut milk and 150ml water and bring to a simmer. Stir in the cavolo nero with a pinch of salt, then sit the chicken thighs on top of the curry, cover with a lid and simmer gently for 15 minutes, stirring occasionally. Remove the pan from the heat.

Immediately before serving, shred the chicken using two forks or roughly chop it into strips and stir it back through the curry. Serve with a dash of paprika to finish.

Substitutions

Cavolo nero: spring greens, spinach or hispi cabbage

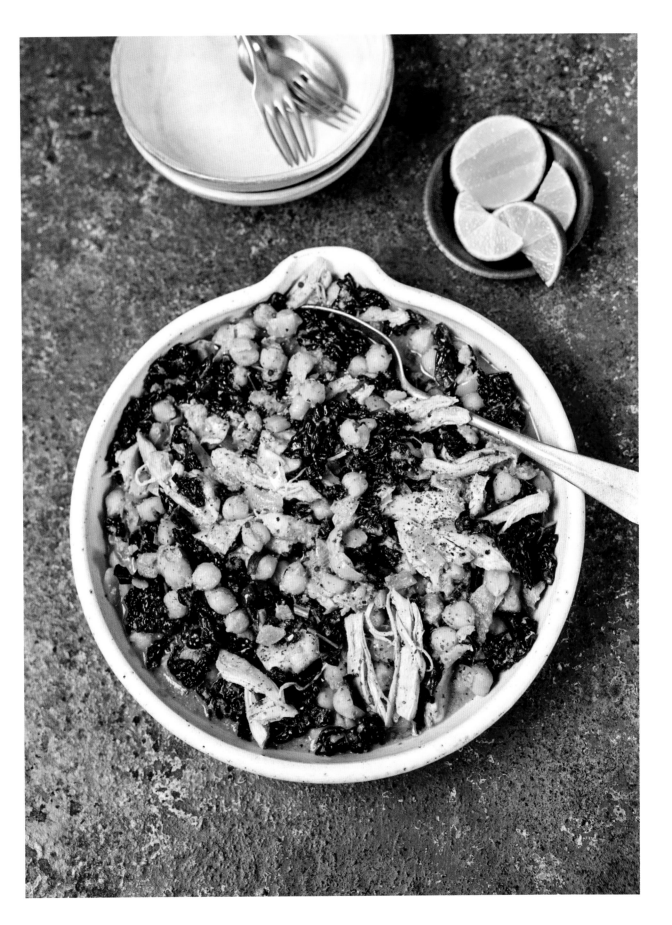

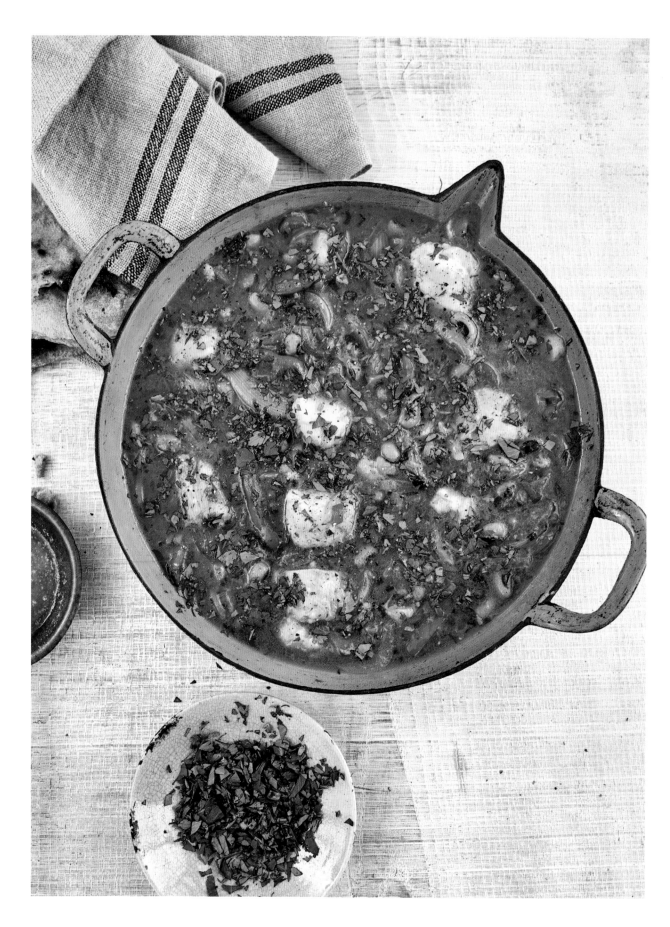

BLACK-EYED BEAN & SNAPPER STEW WITH ROTI

Serves 2

Prep time: 20 minutes
Cook time: 35 minutes

This is a fresh, fragrant and tasty bowl of real comfort food with a delicious mix of spices, delivering all those anti-inflammatory benefits associated with good gut health. To make this vegetarian, simply omit the fish.

2 tbsp coconut oil

1 onion (180g), sliced

1 red pepper (160g), deseeded and sliced

3 garlic cloves, grated

30g fresh ginger, cut into thin matchsticks or grated

1 Scotch bonnet or red chilli, deseeded and finely chopped

6 sprigs of thyme, leaves only

2 tsp medium curry powder

½ tsp ground allspice

Small bunch each of parsley and coriander, stalks and leaves separated and roughly chopped

1 x 400g can black-eyed beans

1 x 400ml can coconut milk

200g skinless red snapper, cut into thick chunks

For the roti

200g wholemeal self-raising flour (or 200g atta and ½ tsp baking powder)

½ tsp salt

120ml warm water

25g butter, melted, or cold-pressed rapeseed oil for a dairy-free version)

Heat the oil in a saucepan over a medium heat. Add the onion and pepper and fry gently for 6 to 7 minutes until softened. Add the garlic, ginger, chilli, thyme, spices, parsley and coriander stalks and fry for 2 minutes.

Drain and rinse the beans, then add them to the pan and pour in the coconut milk and 100ml water. Bring everything to a simmer, season to taste and cook for 15 minutes until thickened. Lower the snapper pieces into the simmering sauce, cover with a lid and cook for 8 minutes until the fish is cooked through.

Meanwhile, to make the roti, combine the flour and salt in a bowl and stir in the water to form a rough dough. Tip out onto a clean work surface and knead for 2 to 3 minutes to make a smooth ball. Divide the dough into 4 equal balls then roll each piece into a thin circle, roughly 20cm in diameter and the thickness of a 20 pence coin (2mm).

Set a dry frying pan over a high heat, add one of the roti and cook for 1 to 2 minutes on each side until lightly blistered. As the roti cooks, press down with a spatula occasionally; it helps to force the steam through the dough and make the roti puff up. Wrap the cooked roti in a clean, dry tea towel once cooked. Brush with the melted butter or oil just before serving.

Remove the stew from the heat, scatter over the chopped herb leaves and serve with the warm roti.

Substitutions

Red snapper: seabass, cod, pollock, hake or monkfish

Thyme: 1 tsp dried thyme or mixed herbs

SOUTH INDIAN-STYLE MONKFISH & LENTIL CURRY

Serves 4

Prep time: 20 minutes
Cook time: 35 minutes

This authentic flavour combination of fresh tomatoes, mustard seeds and curry leaves takes me back to my travels to Kerala and Goa. The addition of lentils and green beans to the tomatoes really packs in the protein and vegetables per portion, making this beautifully balanced and light. Because of the lentils, I don't think this curry needs to be served with rice, but you can if you wish.

2 tbsp coconut oil

1 whole star anise

2 tsp cumin seeds

2 tsp black mustard seeds

1 tsp ground turmeric

12 curry leaves (optional)

150g red lentils, thoroughly washed

1 x 400ml can coconut milk

300ml fish or vegetable stock

600g monkfish, cut into 4cm pieces

300g green beans, halved

150g spinach, roughly chopped

For the curry paste

3 dried Kashmiri chillies, stems removed (or 2 tsp chilli flakes)

2 tbsp desiccated coconut

100ml boiling water

100g red onion, chopped

3 tomatoes (300g), chopped

6 garlic cloves, peeled

25g fresh ginger, roughly chopped

½ tsp each of salt and pepper

To serve

Small bunch of coriander, roughly chopped

2 limes, cut into wedges

For the curry paste, soak the dried chillies and coconut in the boiling water for 10 minutes. Tip the soaked chillies and coconut, along with the water, into a food processor or blender with the remaining ingredients and blend until smooth.

Heat the coconut oil in a heavy-based saucepan over a medium-low heat. Add the star anise, cumin and mustard seeds, turmeric, curry leaves, if using, with seasoning, and fry for 1 to 2 minutes. Add the curry paste and fry for 5 minutes, stirring continuously, until it thickens and intensifies in flavour.

Add the lentils, coconut milk and stock. Bring to a simmer and cook gently for 20 minutes until the lentils are soft.

Add the monkfish, green beans and spinach and cook for a further 8 minutes or until the monkfish is just cooked through.

To serve, spoon the curry into bowls, scatter over the chopped coriander and garnish with lime wedges for squeezing.

Substitutions

Monkfish: prawns or cod loin. Alternatively, to make it vegetarian, swap the monkfish for an extra 200g lentils

Curry paste: cheat by using a shop-bought Keralan curry paste

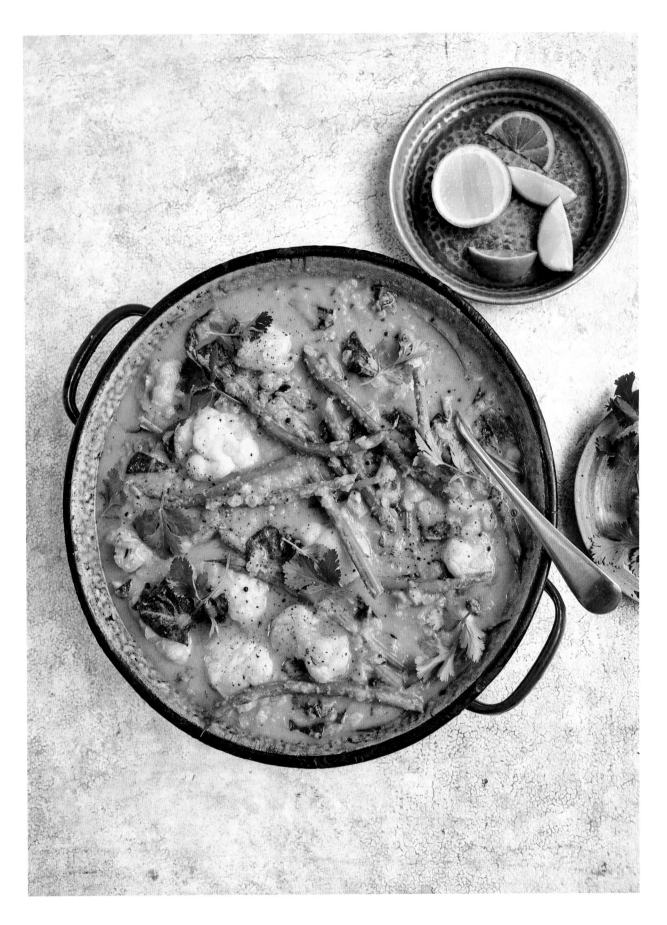

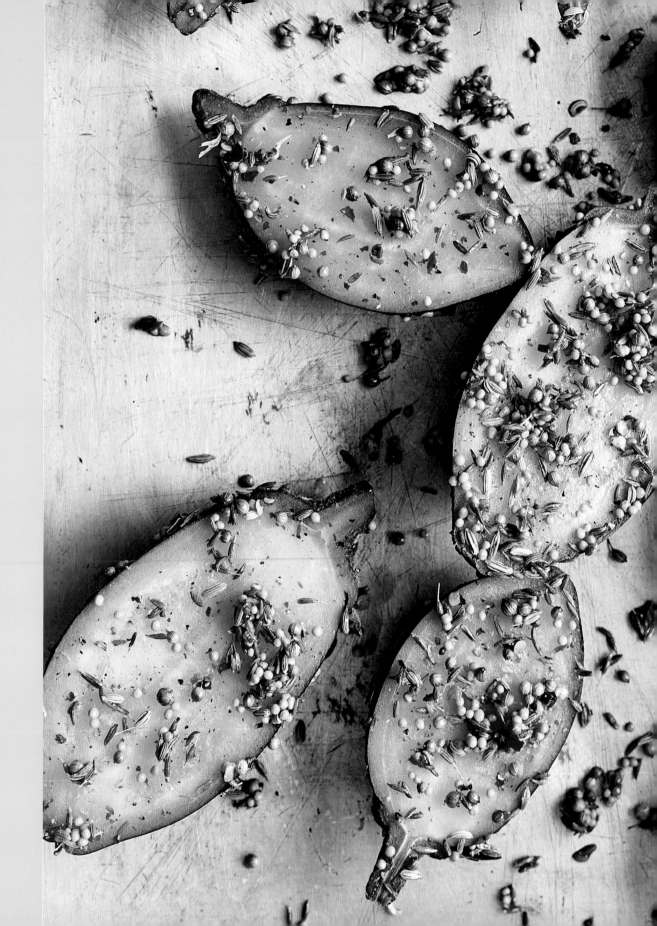

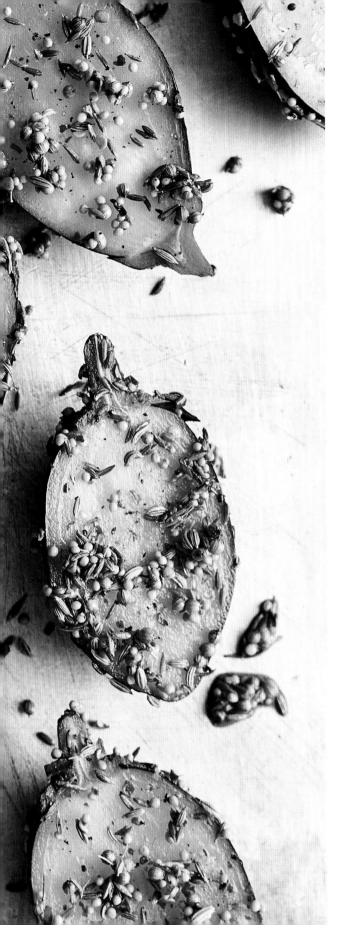

HEALTHY FEASTS

EXPRESS INDIAN FEAST

I've used this formula for a healthy Indian dinner party meal many times and it is super-straightforward. Your guests will be enjoying over three portions of vegetables, a healthy amount of spice and an array of delicious textures and elements – heat from the prawns, tang from the cabbage pickle and creamy cooling yoghurt. Make the curry sauce in advance and then add the prawns to the simmering pan when your guests arrive. You can also prepare the potatoes ahead of time, mixing them in the spices and oil, ready to roast before serving. Allow about 90 minutes in total to cook this entire feast. Start with the potatoes and prawns, then move onto the pickle and raita.

GUNPOWDER POTATOES

3 tbsp **avocado oil** or **olive oil**

2 tsp **fennel seeds**

2 tsp **cumin seeds**

2 tsp **black mustard seeds**

1 tsp **ground turmeric**

30g **fresh ginger**, julienned

600g **new potatoes**, quartered

10g **coriander**, chopped

Serves 5 to 6

Prep time: 5 minutes
Cook time: 45 minutes

Preheat the oven to 200°C fan and warm a large roasting tin for a few minutes.

Pour the oil for the potatoes into the tin, stir in the spices and ginger, then add the potatoes and a good pinch of salt and stir to coat. Roast for 40 to 45 minutes, giving everything a shake occasionally, until crisp. Top with coriander before serving, then transfer to a serving bowl.

CUCUMBER RAITA

½ **cucumber** (200g), grated

300g **natural yoghurt** or **coconut yoghurt**

½ tsp **garam masala**

Serves 5 to 6

Prep time: 5 minutes

Coarsely grate the cucumber onto a clean tea towel and squeeze out as much excess liquid as possible. Tip into a bowl, stir in the yoghurt and garam masala and season well.

2 tbsp **avocado oil** or **olive oil**

1 **onion** (180g), thinly sliced

30g **fresh ginger**, grated

5 **garlic cloves**, grated

2 tsp **black mustard seeds**

1 tbsp **mild curry powder** or **garam masala**

700g **baby tomatoes**, roughly chopped

2 tbsp **tomato purée**

400g **baby leaf spinach**

500g **raw jumbo prawns**, shelled and deveined

10g **coriander**, chopped

2 tsp **dried fenugreek leaves** (optional)

PRAWN MASALA CURRY

Serves 5 to 6

Prep time: 15 minutes
Cook time: 45 minutes

Heat the oil in a wide pan over a medium-high heat. Add the onion, ginger and garlic with the spices and a little salt, and fry for 8 minutes until the onion has softened. Tip in the tomatoes and tomato purée, cover and cook for 25 to 30 minutes until the tomatoes have broken down.

Stir in the spinach, a handful at a time until wilted. When the sauce is simmering, stir in the prawns, cover and cook for 5 to 6 minutes until all the prawns are cooked through. Serve with chopped coriander and dried fenugreek leaves, if using, stirred through.

1 small **red cabbage** (400g), core removed and finely shredded

150ml **white wine vinegar**

150ml **hot water**

1 tbsp **soft light brown sugar**

1 tbsp **fennel seeds**

1 tsp **fine salt**

QUICK RED CABBAGE PICKLE

Serves 5 to 6

Prep time: 10 minutes, plus pickling time
Cook time: 5 minutes

Tip the shredded cabbage into a large heatproof bowl.

Combine the remaining ingredients in a saucepan and bring to the boil, stirring until the sugar and salt have dissolved. Pour over the cabbage, stir for a minute or two then set aside to cool completely. It should only take 30 minutes but the longer you leave it the better. Drain the liquid and squeeze out any excess before serving in a large bowl.

Photographed overleaf...

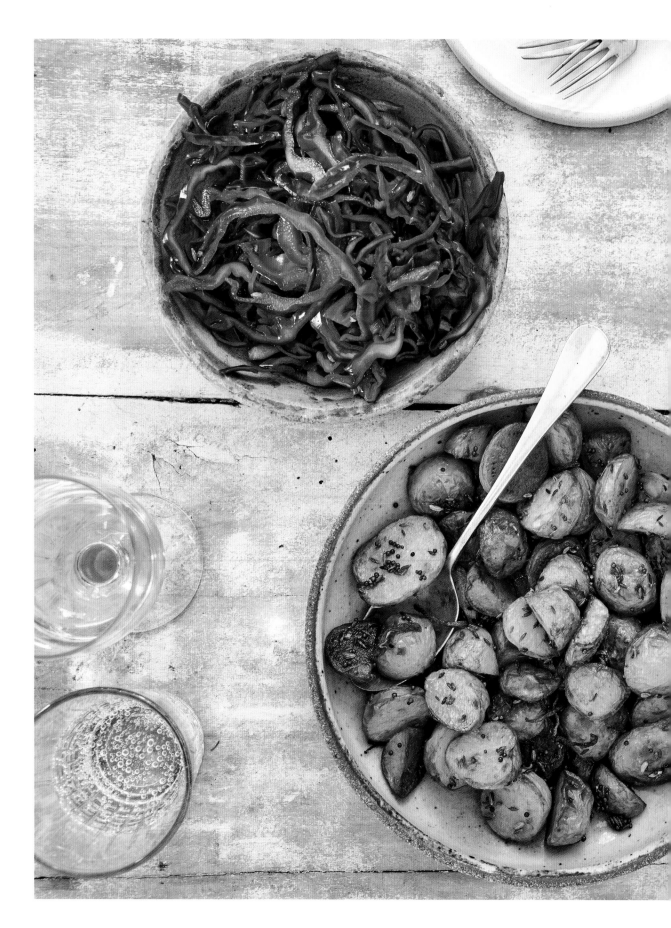

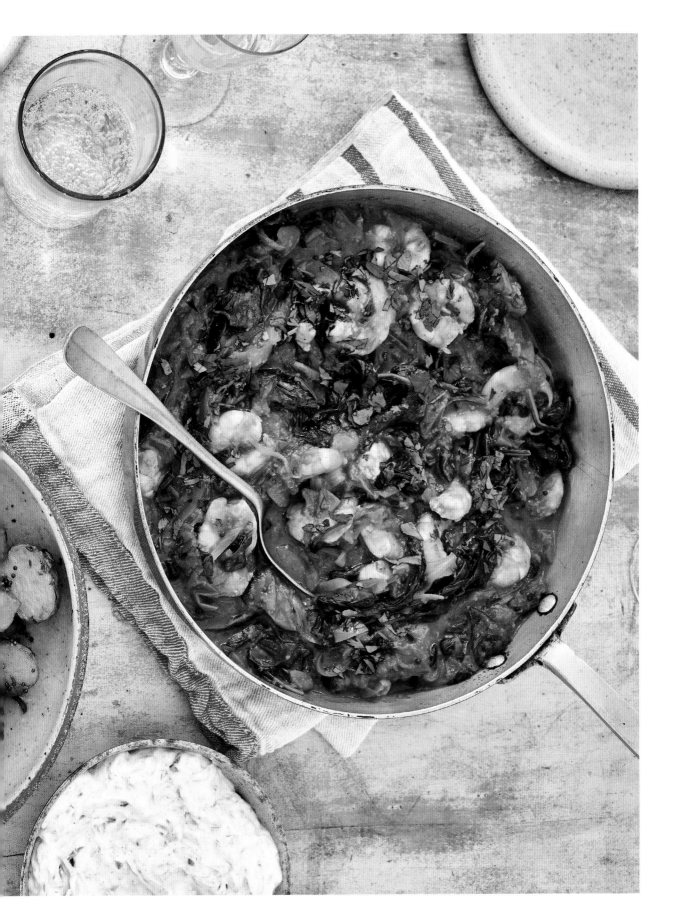

'TAKE ME TO KOREA' DINNER PARTY

This is pretty inauthentic for a Korean feast, but it is super-adventurous and healthy while being delicious and easy to prepare. The rice I use is high-fibre and fantastic for absorbing all the flavours from the sweet and spicy sauces. The spicy beans are a revelation in the marinade, and the simple greens are elevated by the sesame dressing. Bring all the elements together for a dinner party by serving the rice, beans and greens with the dipping sauce, some kimchi and a few sheets of seaweed. It will only take 1 hour in total to bring everything together. Perfect for an adventurous, healthy feast.

400g short-grain brown rice, thoroughly rinsed

600ml boiling water

2 tbsp rice vinegar

1 tbsp mirin

RICE

Serves 5 to 6

Prep time: 5 minutes
Cook time: 30 minutes

Tip the rice into a pan over a medium heat and toast the grains for 1 minute. Add the boiling water and bring to a gentle simmer. Cover and cook for 20 minutes, then take off the heat, let stand for 10 minutes. Stir through the vinegar, mirin and salt to taste, then cover again with the lid to keep warm.

3 tbsp tamari or **soy sauce**

2 tbsp rice vinegar

2 tbsp tahini

1 tbsp toasted sesame seeds

600g spring greens, stalks removed, leaves roughly shredded

SESAME GREENS

Serves 5 to 6

Prep time: 5 minutes
Cook time: 5 minutes

Whisk the tamari or soy sauce, vinegar, tahini and sesame seeds together in a large serving bowl and set aside. Bring a large pan of water to the boil, add the greens and blanch for 2 to 3 minutes. Drain thoroughly then tip into the bowl with the dressing and toss to coat.

3 tbsp **tamari or soy sauce**

2 tbsp **gochujang**

2 tbsp **rice vinegar**

2 tsp **soft light brown sugar**

2 tsp **toasted sesame seeds**

2 tbsp **sesame oil**

1 tbsp **hot water**

400g green beans, roughly chopped

3 garlic cloves, grated

2 x 400g cans kidney beans, drained and rinsed

for the dipping sauce

2 tbsp **gochujang**

2 tbsp **tamari** or **soy sauce**

2 tbsp **rice vinegar**

1 tbsp **doenjang** or **white miso paste**

1 tbsp **maple syrup**

1 **garlic clove**, grated

4 spring onions, finely chopped

to serve

100g kimchi

10g toasted nori sheets

Note

If you stick with tamari rather than soy sauce, then the whole feast is plant-based, gluten-free and nut-free. Just check the labels on all the store-bought ingredients.

SWEET SPICY BEANS

Serves 5 to 6

Prep time: 5 minutes
Cook time: 20 minutes

Whisk the tamari or soy sauce, gochujang, vinegar, sugar, sesame seeds, 1 tablespoon of the sesame oil and the water together in a small bowl and set aside.

Heat the remaining tablespoon of sesame oil in a wok over medium heat, then add the green beans and stir-fry for 2 to 3 minutes. Add the garlic, fry for a further 2 minutes then stir in the kidney beans. Cook for another minute then stir in the sauce and let everything bubble up. Cover and cook over a low heat for 10 minutes (if it gets too dry, splash in some extra water) then take off the heat.

TO SERVE

Combine the ingredients for the dipping sauce in a small bowl and stir until smooth.

Bring all the elements together on the table and allow everyone to tuck in.

Photographed overleaf...

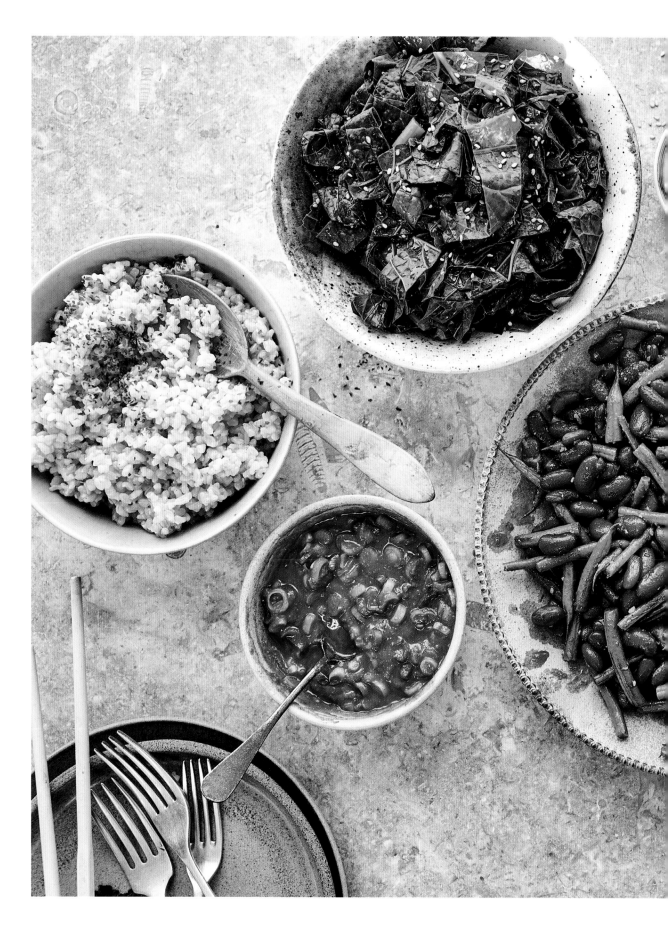

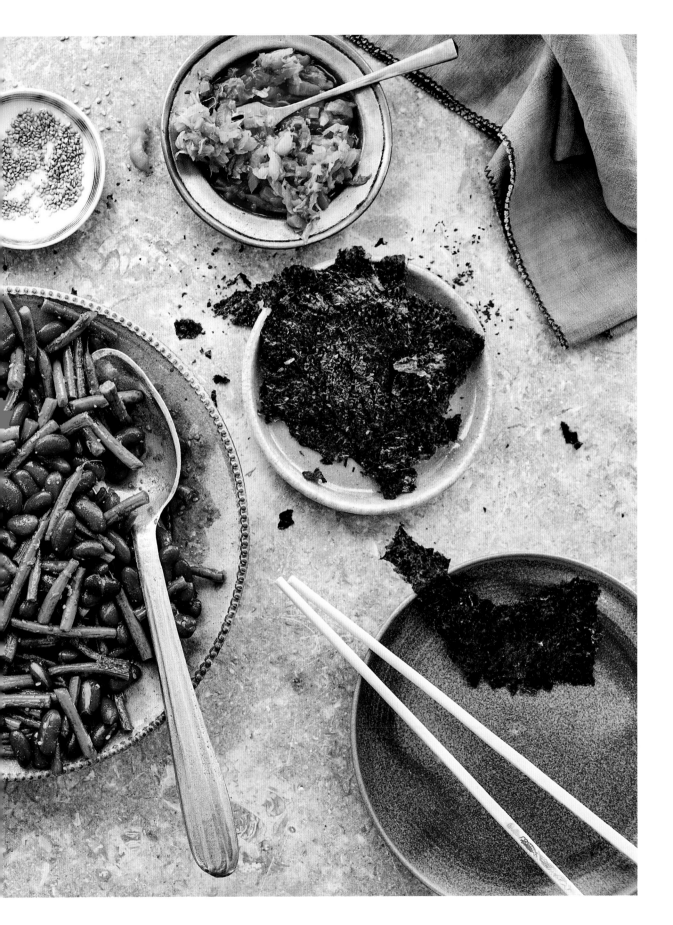

EXPRESS MIDDLE EASTERN FEAST

This feast has a great mixture of flavours, good serving sizes, and a fantastic mix of vegetables that bring a spectacular visual appeal to the meal. Perfect for a dinner party or big family dinner that everyone will enjoy, plus it's packed with vegetables and plant diversity to support wellbeing. Just 90 minutes is all you need to conjure up this spectacular collection of dishes.

2 x 400g cans chickpeas, drained and rinsed

2 tbsp tahini

2 tbsp extra virgin olive oil, plus extra to serve

Juice of 2 lemons

1 garlic clove, grated

1 tsp ground cumin

1 tsp sumac

CHEAT'S HUMMUS

Serves 5 to 6

Prep time: 5 minutes
Cook time: 5 minutes

Tip the chickpeas into a saucepan over a medium heat with a little boiling water, to warm through for 5 minutes. Drain then add to a food processor with the tahini, olive oil, lemon juice, garlic and cumin. Blend until smooth, gradually adding ice-cold water until you have a silky-smooth paste. Season with a pinch of salt then spread out on a serving platter. Drizzle with more olive oil and sprinkle over the sumac.

1 onion (180g), thinly sliced

1 large fennel bulb (300g), thinly sliced

300g new potatoes, thinly sliced

2 tbsp extra virgin olive oil

10–12 sardine fillets or **6 whole sardines**

1 tbsp za'atar, plus extra to serve

Finely grated zest and juice of 1 lemon

Pinch of chilli powder

Small bunch of parsley, finely chopped

Small bunch of dill, finely chopped

ZA'ATAR GRILLED SARDINES

Serves 5 to 6

Prep time: 15 minutes
Cook time: 40 minutes

Preheat the oven to 200°C fan. Tip the onion, fennel and potatoes into a roasting tin. Drizzle over the olive oil, season well, toss to coat and roast for 30 minutes until soft. Preheat the grill to high, toss the sardines in the za'atar, season well and lay over the top of the vegetables. Grill for 4 to 5 minutes until the fish skin is lightly charred and blistered. Transfer to a serving platter and top with a generous pinch of za'atar, the lemon zest and chilli powder. Just before serving, scatter over the parsley and dill, with the lemon juice.

300g watercress

300g rocket

Finely grated zest of 2 lemons

Juice of 1 lemon

2 tbsp extra virgin olive oil

50g pistachios, finely chopped

LEMON PISTACHIO GREENS

Serves 5 to 6

Prep time: 5 minutes
Cook time: 5 minutes

Bring a saucepan of salted water to the boil, add the watercress and rocket and blanch for 30 seconds. Drain, rinse under cold running water then plunge into a bowl of iced water. Squeeze out as much water as possible, then transfer to a large bowl. Add the lemon zest, juice and olive oil and season well. Toss to combine then transfer to a platter and top with the pistachios.

800g mixed peppers, deseeded and cut into thick wedges

3 tbsp extra virgin olive oil

2 tbsp pomegranate molasses

MOLASSES-ROAST PEPPERS

Serves 5 to 6

Prep time: 5 minutes
Cook time: 40 minutes

Preheat the oven to 200°C fan. Tip the peppers into a roasting tin, drizzle with the oil and season. Roast for 40 minutes until soft and blistered, giving them a stir a couple of times during cooking. To finish, drizzle over the pomegranate molasses and toss to combine. Spread out on a serving platter and set aside.

2 large aubergines (800g), cut into 3cm thick wedges

3 tbsp harissa paste

2 tbsp extra virgin olive oil

100g rocket

HARISSA-ROAST AUBERGINES

Serves 5 to 6

Prep time: 5 minutes
Cook time: 40 minutes

Tip the aubergines into another roasting tin and coat with the harissa and olive oil. Season with salt and pepper and cook alongside the peppers for 40 minutes at 200°C fan. Spoon the aubergines onto a platter with rocket leaves just before serving.

Photographed overleaf...

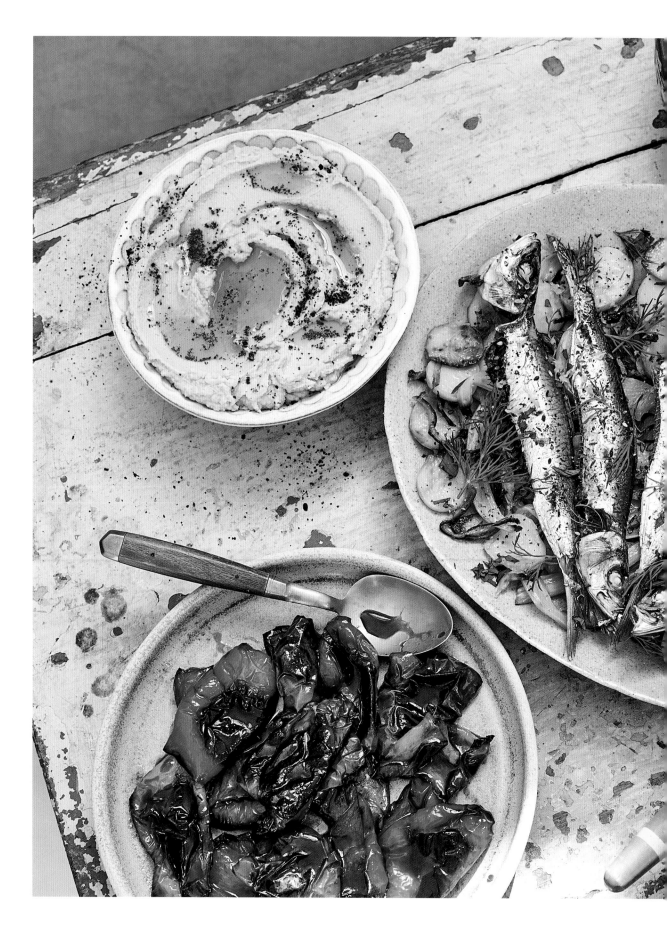

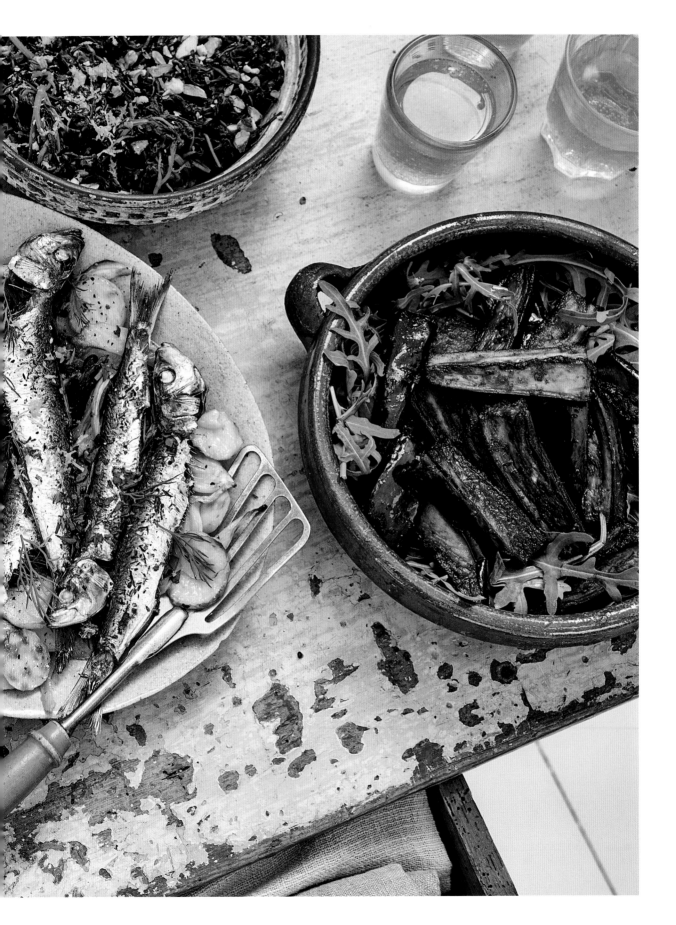

EXPRESS VEGAN DINNER PARTY

I love one of the recipe tester's comments on this meal: "It was amazing food that looked like you'd been in the kitchen all day when in reality the prep took no time at all!" That's exactly how a feast should be. A great selection of food that's nourishing and authentic, as well as minimal stress so you can enjoy one of the best lifestyle hacks for health: connection. This masala-baked cauliflower centrepiece with aubergines, ginger and turmeric dal with saag, coconut yoghurt is a beautiful collection of complex flavours and, trust me, nobody realises it's fully plant-based.

3 tsp garam masala

2 tsp paprika

1 tsp ground turmeric

4 tbsp olive oil

1 large cauliflower (750g), quartered, leaves removed, roughly chopped

MASALA-BAKED CAULIFLOWER

Serves 5 to 6

Prep time: 5 minutes
Cook time: 40 minutes

Preheat the oven to 200°C fan.

Mix the spices and oil in a bowl with plenty of seasoning. Brush onto the cauliflower quarters and leaves, adding a little more oil if needed. Bake in the oven for 35 to 40 minutes until golden, turning the cauliflower and ruffling the leaves halfway through.

500g baby aubergines, halved lengthways

2 tsp coriander seeds

2 tsp cumin seeds

2 tsp mustard seeds

1 tsp fennel seeds

1 tsp chilli flakes

½ tsp black pepper

4 tbsp olive oil

BAKED AUBERGINES IN SPICED OIL

Serves 5 to 6

Prep time: 5 minutes
Cook time: 35 minutes

Preheat the oven to 200°C fan.

Mix the aubergines, spices and oil in a roasting tin, coating the aubergine pieces well. Sprinkle with plenty of salt and bake in the oven for 30 to 35 minutes until golden.

GINGER & TURMERIC DAL

2 tbsp coconut oil

40g fresh ginger, grated

2 tsp mustard seeds

1 star anise

1 tsp Kashmiri chilli powder (or paprika)

1 tsp ground turmeric

2 tsp cumin seeds

400g red lentils, soaked for 10 minutes then drained

1 vegetable stock cube

1 x 400ml can coconut milk

300ml hot water

200g spinach, roughly chopped

Serves 5 to 6

Prep time: 10 minutes, plus soaking
Cook time: 20 minutes

Melt the coconut oil in a large saucepan over a medium heat. Add the ginger, spices and plenty of seasoning and fry for 2 to 3 minutes. Add the lentils and cook for a further 1 minute. Crumble in the stock cube, pour in the coconut milk and hot water, bring to a simmer and cook for 15 minutes until the lentils are soft, adding more water if necessary to stop it drying out. Add the spinach for the last 2 minutes of cooking to gently wilt.

SPEEDY SAAG

200g spinach, roughly chopped

300g kale, stems removed and roughly chopped

300g spring greens, stems removed and roughly chopped

500ml hot water

For the tarka

4 tbsp avocado oil or coconut oil

12 curry leaves

2 tsp mustard seeds

2 tsp cumin seeds

2 tsp fennel seeds

1 tsp chilli flakes

Serves 5 to 6

Prep time: 5 minutes
Cook time: 25 minutes

Place the chopped spinach, kale and spring greens in a large pan. Add the hot water and plenty of salt and pepper, and simmer for 15 to 20 minutes until broken down. Blend with a stick blender; the mixture should be fairly thick (you can add a tablespoon of coconut yoghurt to thicken, if needed).

Meanwhile, in a small pan over a medium heat, make the tarka (a spiced oil mix). Add the oil, curry leaves, spices and some salt to the pan and cook for a few minutes until the mustard seeds begin to pop. Then throw over the saag in the pan to serve.

TO SERVE

250g coconut yoghurt

Juice of ½ lemon

Pinch of garam masala

Cooked brown basmati rice

Flatbreads

Mango pickle

Whip the coconut yoghurt with the lemon juice and salt to taste and dust with a pinch of garam masala to serve. Serve with brown basmati rice, flatbreads and mango pickle.

Photographed overleaf...

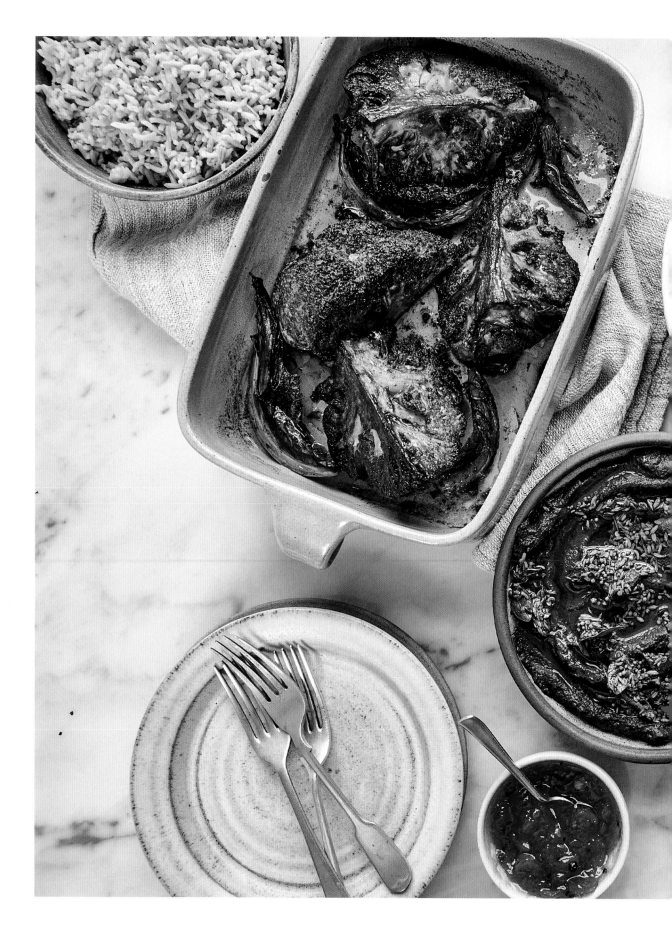

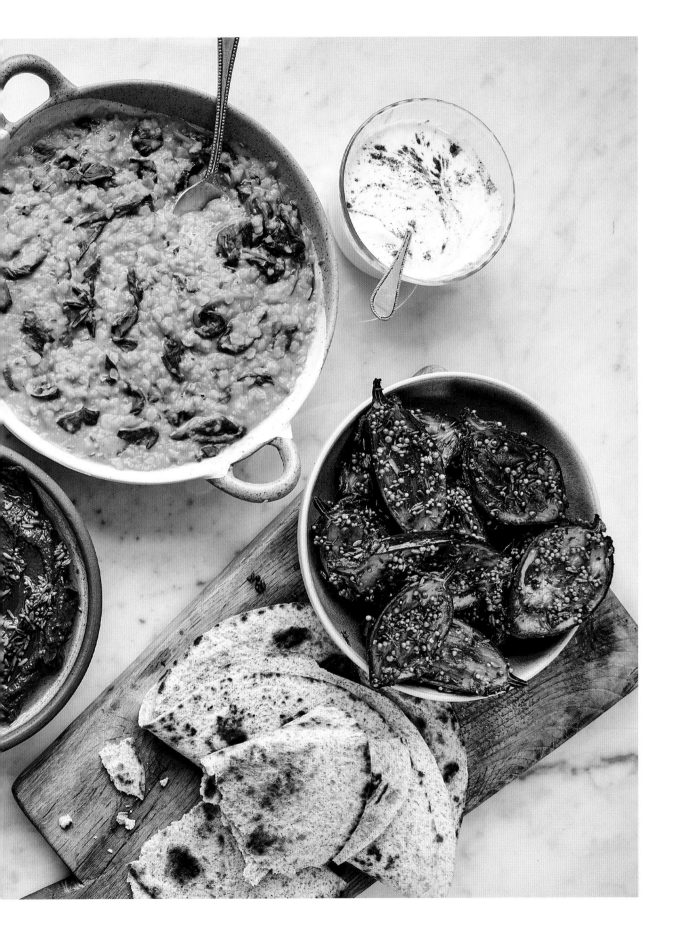

LEBANESE-STYLE CHICKEN TACOS

Serves 4

Prep time: 20 minutes, plus marinating
Cook time: 30 minutes

The combination of Middle Eastern spices and Mexican food might seem inauthentic at first, but actually this has worked well for hundreds of years, and the cultural influence runs deep in Mexico. The Arab diaspora brought their delicious culinary heritage to Mexican cuisine, including the kebab, which I've tried to recreate without the need for a rotating grill! This meal is packed with vegetables, flavour and plenty of diversity, making it healthy and delicious.

750g boneless, skinless chicken thighs

2 tsp sumac

For the marinade

2 tbsp extra virgin olive oil

Juice of 1 lime

1 tbsp baharat spice mix (also known as Lebanese 7-spice)

2 tsp dried oregano

2 garlic cloves, grated

For the cabbage

½ red or white cabbage (300g), shredded

1 tsp salt

1 tsp sugar

2 tsp dried oregano

To make the marinade, put all the ingredients in a bowl with some seasoning. Add the chicken, toss to coat, then cover and chill in the fridge for at least 30 minutes (but 2 hours or more is preferable).

Tip the cabbage into a bowl, add the salt, sugar and oregano and massage for a couple of minutes, using your hands, to soften. Leave in the fridge and discard any water that has been drawn out before serving.

Preheat the grill to high. Lay the chicken on the grill tray in an even layer and grill for 10 minutes on each side or until lightly charred. Remove from the heat and, using two forks, pull apart the chicken, then place it back under the grill to cook for a further 2 minutes. Sprinkle over the sumac and set aside to rest.

For the black beans

1 tbsp olive oil

1 small shallot (80g), diced

1 tsp ground cumin

1 tsp smoked paprika

2 tbsp sun-dried tomato paste

1 x 200g can chopped tomatoes

1 x 400g can black beans, drained and rinsed

Juice of 1 lime

For the chipotle yoghurt

250g natural yoghurt

1–2 tsp chipotle paste, to taste

To serve

8 small soft corn tortillas

2–3 tbsp pickled jalapeños

Small bunch coriander (20g), roughly chopped

2 limes, cut into wedges

Substitutions

Baharat: ras el hanout, shawarma seasoning or za'atar

Chicken: sliced oyster mushrooms or crumbled tempeh to make it vegetarian

While the chicken is cooking, heat the olive oil in a saucepan over a medium heat. Add the shallot with a little seasoning and sauté for 5 minutes. Add the spices and sun-dried tomato paste, stir for 1 minute, then add the chopped tomatoes and beans. Bring to a simmer for 10 minutes, then remove from the heat and stir in the lime juice.

Wrap the corn tortillas in foil and warm in the oven while you get everything ready.

Mix together the yoghurt and chipotle paste. Serve all the dishes family-style at the table with sumac chicken, black beans, cabbage, pickled jalapeños, chopped coriander, lime wedges and chipotle yoghurt in separate dishes, with the warmed tortillas alongside.

Photographed overleaf...

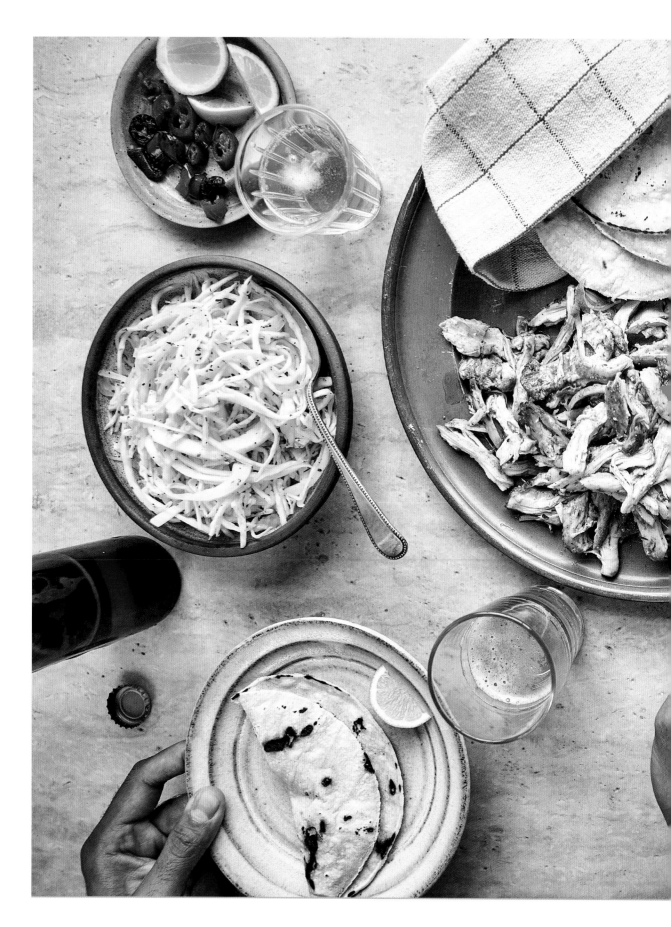

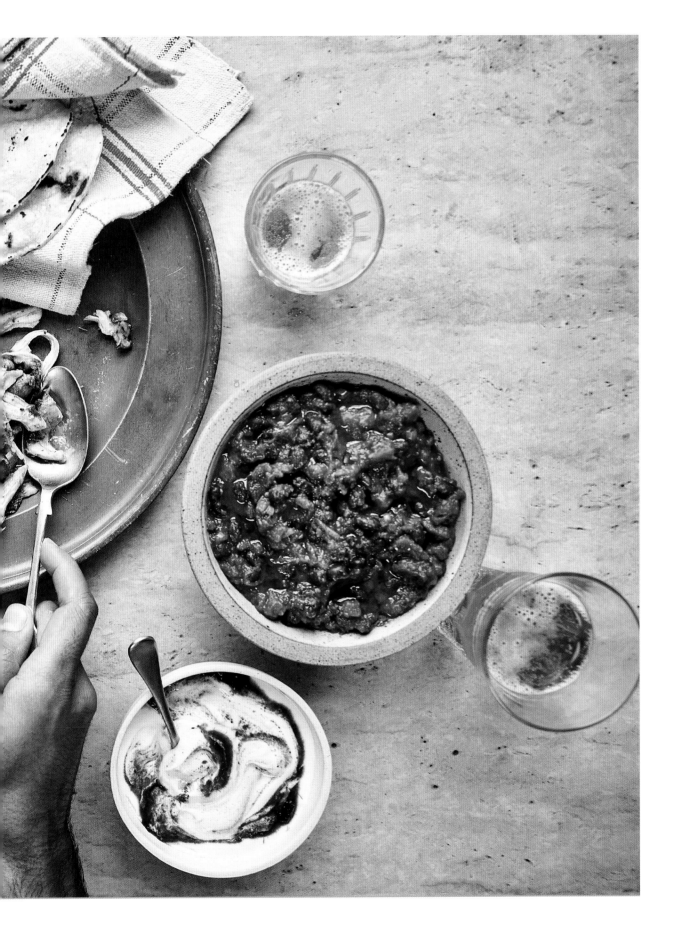

EXPRESS MEDITERRANEAN FEAST

A stress-free baked salmon, some slow-cooked peas and a beautiful big salad – this is how to effortlessly entertain during a family-style lunch or dinner with a group of friends or loved ones. These dishes are all super-simple and, in combination, are a powerhouse of nutrition with buckets of punchy flavour. The savoury sourdough is optional, but it helps to use up bread leftover from the week – and it tastes amazing. You can make all the elements for this feast in about 1 hour 30 minutes and most of the work is done by the oven!

3 tbsp extra virgin olive oil

200g shallots, diced

8 garlic cloves, sliced

200g fennel, diced

10g sage, stalks tied to keep the bunch together

1 tsp white miso paste

2 tsp caraway seeds

2 tsp nigella seeds

250g dried split green peas, soaked for 30 minutes then drained

500ml vegetable stock

200g frozen spinach, defrosted

For the dressing

10g parsley, stalks and leaves finely chopped

3 tbsp red wine vinegar

6 tbsp extra virgin olive oil

2 tsp capers

2 tsp wholegrain mustard

Substitutions

Miso paste: 2 anchovy fillets in oil

SPLIT GREEN PEA STEW WITH SAGE

Serves 6

Prep time: 30 minutes
Cook time: 50 minutes

Heat the oil in a large flameproof casserole dish over a medium heat. Add the shallot, garlic and fennel and sauté for 8 minutes, until softened and starting to colour. Stir the tied sage into the vegetables with the miso paste and caraway and nigella seeds. Cook for a further 2 minutes before adding the drained split peas.

Stir the peas in the pan for 2 minutes. Add the stock, bring to a simmer with the lid on the pan and cook for 35 minutes or until the peas are tender but not mushy. The pan contents should be slightly wet and not completely dry; if needed, add a touch more boiling water. Throw the spinach into the pan for the last 10 minutes of the cooking time and allow to heat through.

Meanwhile, whisk together all the ingredients for the dressing in a small bowl, then season to taste.

Give everything a stir, then remove the pan from the heat. Remove the sage and finish the stew with the dressing.

1 x 800g–1kg salmon fillet, pin-boned and scaled

3 tbsp olive oil

2 tbsp red wine vinegar

6 garlic cloves, grated

2 rosemary sprigs, leaves chopped

1 lemon, cut into wedges

For the pangrattato

2 slices rye bread (can be stale)

1 garlic clove, grated

1 rosemary sprig, leaves finely chopped

3 tbsp olive oil

Finely grated zest of ½ lemon

BAKED ROSEMARY & GARLIC SALMON WITH PANGRATTATO

Serves 6

Prep time: 10 minutes, plus marinating
Cook time: 15 minutes

Preheat the oven to 200°C fan.

Place the salmon on a large baking tray and smother with the olive oil, vinegar, garlic, rosemary and plenty of seasoning. (If you have time to marinate the fish, 1 hour would be ideal.) Bake in the oven for 15 minutes or until the salmon flakes easily and is nicely coloured on top.

Meanwhile, crumble the rye bread slices by hand into a dry pan over a medium heat, then break it up further into fine pieces in the pan with a wooden spoon. Dry-fry for 2 to 3 minutes until smelling toasty, then add the garlic and rosemary and gradually pour in the oil to crisp up in the pan. Stir for 2 to 3 minutes then set aside to cool. Toss through the lemon zest and scatter over the baked salmon.

200g watercress, roughly chopped

200g radicchio leaves, some torn, some chopped

150g baby gem leaves, roughly chopped

60g pumpkin seeds, toasted and roughly chopped

For the dressing

10g parsley, finely chopped

10g chives, finely chopped

Juice of 1 lemon

1 tsp wholegrain mustard

1 garlic clove, grated

2 tbsp natural yoghurt

1 anchovy fillet in oil (optional)

5 tbsp extra virgin olive oil

WATERCRESS, RADICCHIO & LETTUCE SALAD WITH HERBY GREEN DRESSING

Serves 6

Prep time: 15 minutes

Put the watercress, radicchio and baby gem leaves in a large salad bowl.

To make the dressing, put the parsley, chives and lemon juice in a small food processor, then add the mustard, garlic, yoghurt and anchovy fillet, if using. Blitz until smooth, gradually pouring in the olive oil as you blend. Taste and season according to your preference.

To serve, toss the dressing through the leaves and scatter the pumpkin seeds on top.

Photographed on pages 232-3

250g sourdough bread, roughly torn into 3cm chunks

1 sweet potato (240g), peeled and thinly sliced

1 red onion (180g), thinly sliced

2 tbsp olive oil

600ml almond milk

2 tsp cornflour

3 tsp dried tarragon

30g pumpkin seeds

For the kale pesto (optional)

30g walnuts, crumbled

1 garlic clove, crushed

100g kale, stalks removed, leaves roughly torn

Bunch of basil, leaves only

Finely grated zest of 1 lemon and **a squeeze of juice**

180–200ml olive oil

SAVOURY SOURDOUGH PUDDING WITH KALE PESTO

Serves 6

Prep time: 20 minutes
Cook time: 1 hour 10 minutes

Preheat the oven to 180°C fan.

Tip the sourdough bread, sweet potato and onion into an ovenproof dish, drizzle over the oil and give everything a good mix. Bake in the oven for 30 minutes, stirring halfway through the cooking time, until the vegetables have started to soften and the bread is crisp.

Whisk the almond milk, cornflour, dried tarragon and a pinch of salt and pepper together in a jug, then pour over the bread and vegetables. Stir everything together, then scatter over the pumpkin seeds. Return to the oven for 40 minutes or until the top is golden and the liquid is just set, with a slight wobble. Leave to stand for 5 minutes.

For the pesto, if making, put the walnuts, garlic, kale, basil and lemon zest into a food processor and blend, gradually adding the oil, until you have a smooth, vibrant green pesto. Add a squeeze of lemon juice and season to taste with a pinch of salt. (You can buy good-quality store-bought pesto, but freshly made is delicious.)

TO SERVE

Bring all the elements together on the table and allow everyone to serve themselves.

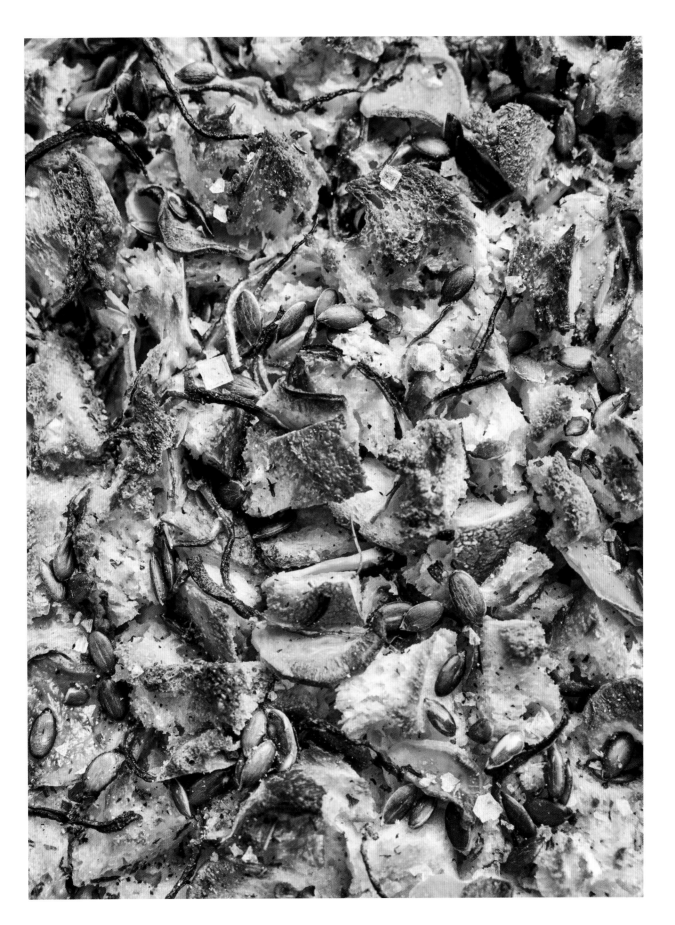

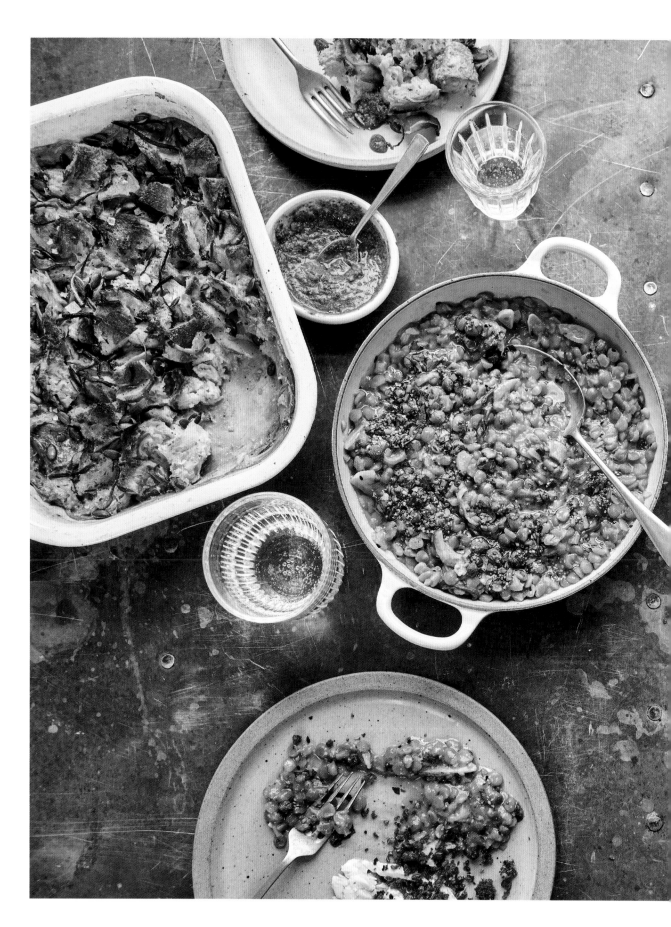

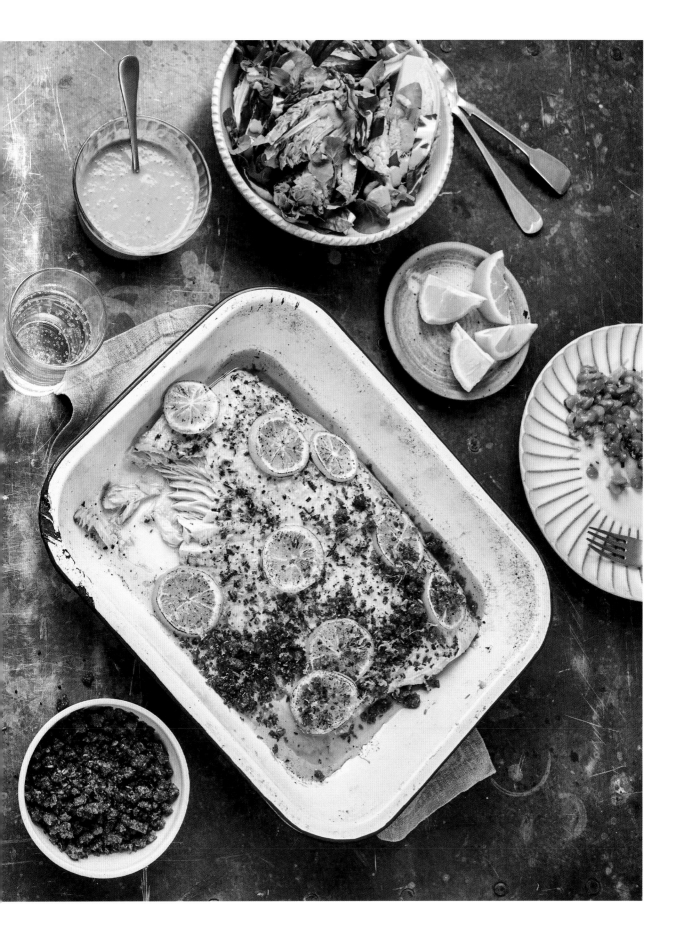

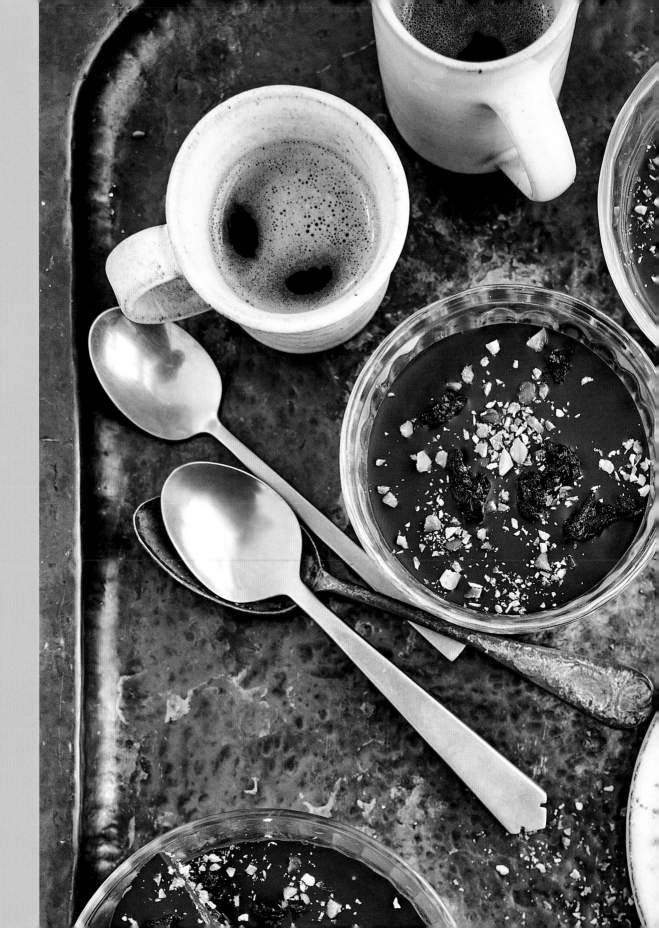

SWEET

APPLE & PEAR CRUMBLE WITH MISO & VANILLA

Serves 4

Prep time: 15 minutes
Cook time: 25 minutes

This sweet-salty dessert is a glorious twist on a classic dish. The miso combination with apples and pears delivers a beautiful salted-caramel flavour and brings out the natural sweetness of these humble fruits. Serve as it is, or with vanilla ice cream, cream or coconut yoghurt.

2–3 pears (500g), peeled, cored and diced

3 Bramley apples (600g), peeled, cored and diced

Juice of 1 lemon

2 tbsp coconut sugar

1 tbsp white miso paste

1 vanilla pod, split lengthways and seeds scraped (or 2 tsp vanilla extract or paste)

For the crumble topping

75g oats (gluten-free, if necessary)

75g ground almonds

2 tbsp coconut oil

2 tbsp coconut sugar

To serve

Cream, **vanilla ice cream** or **coconut yoghurt**

Preheat the oven to 180°C fan.

Combine the pears, apples, lemon juice, sugar, miso paste and vanilla seeds in a flameproof casserole. Set over a medium heat, cover with a lid and cook for 5 minutes until the fruit begins to soften.

Meanwhile, combine the topping ingredients in a bowl with a pinch of salt and work everything with your fingertips until the mixture begins to clump together.

Scatter the crumble topping over the fruit in an even layer, then transfer to the oven and bake for 15 minutes until golden brown. Leave to stand for 5 minutes before serving.

Substitutions

Coconut sugar: white or brown sugar

Coconut oil: any neutral oil, such as cold-pressed rapeseed

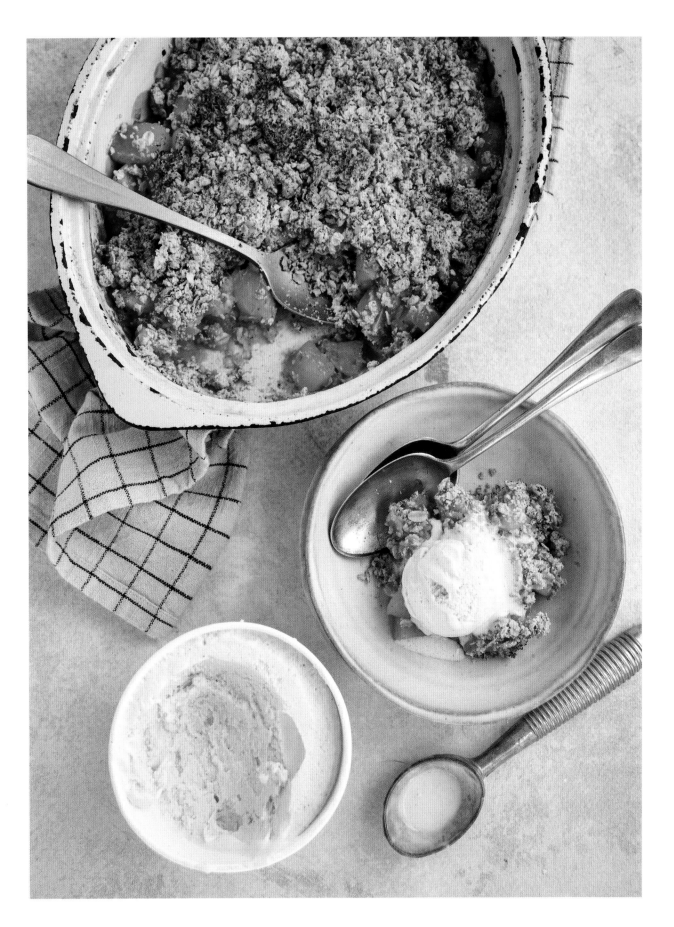

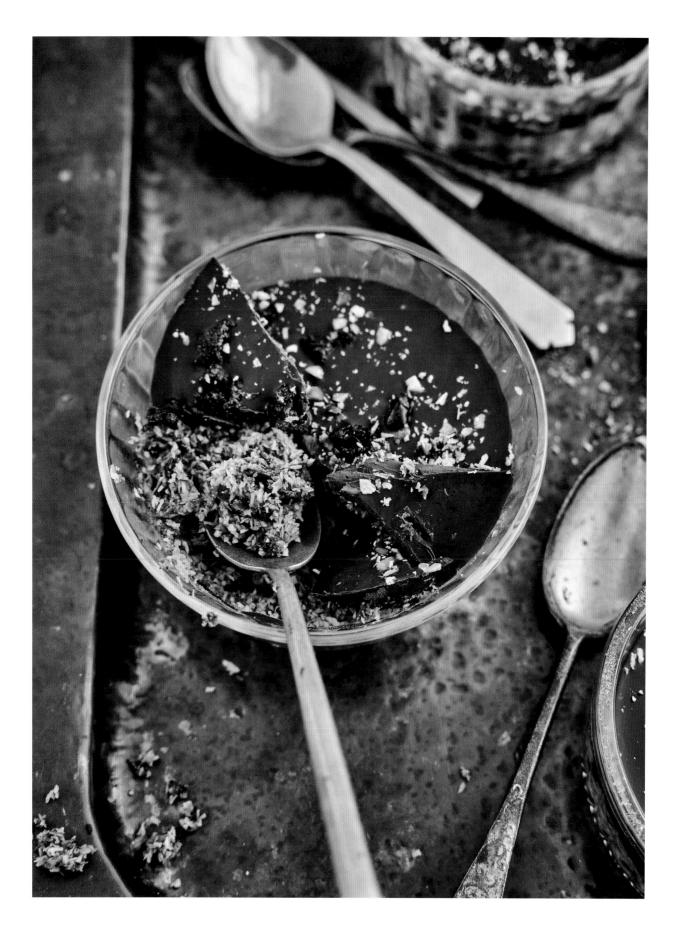

DECONSTRUCTED CHERRY RIPES

Serves 6

Prep time: 30 minutes, plus chilling

My favorite Aussie chocolate bar is a cherry ripe. The coconut, chocolate and cherry combination echoes my preferred baked item as well, the lamington. This recipe is super-simple to make and has all the elements of both these indulgent sweets. As far as a sweet treat goes, this hits all the points for me.

250g cherries, stoned

140g dessicated coconut

30g date molasses or **maple syrup**

30g dried cherries, finely chopped

100g dark chocolate, 80% cocoa solids, roughly chopped

15g pistachios, finely chopped

Roughly blend the cherries in a blender and strain through a fine sieve. (Keep the juice to drink as a cherry shot later as a reward for your efforts.)

In a large mixing bowl, using your hands, mix the blended cherries with the coconut, date molasses or syrup, and two-thirds of the dried cherries. Bring it together until the mixture is combined and feels firm. If it feels too crumbly, add some of the reserved cherry juice.

Divide the mixture evenly between 6 freezer-safe ramekins or small bowls and press down firmly, creating a flat top so that none of the chocolate will be able to seep through the mixture.

Melt the chocolate in a heatproof bowl set over a pan of gently simmering water, making sure the base of the bowl is not touching the water. Spoon the melted chocolate into the ramekins, creating a flat layer on top of the cherry mixture.

Sprinkle over the remaining dried cherries and the pistachios, then immediately transfer to the fridge to cool until set, about 45 to 60 minutes.

Crack into the ramekins with spoons and enjoy as a sweet treat.

GRANITAS

With their sharp, sour flavour combinations, these granitas are refreshing. You could serve them as a palate cleanser or a summer treat. The hint of cardamom with pistachios is a favourite childhood flavour combination that transports me back to Indian summers. Delicious and simple. When you are trying to increase the diversity of plant-based foods in your diet, these recipes include things you perhaps wouldn't normally consider, but are sure to enjoy!

250g pomegranate seeds

Juice of 2 limes

1 tsp soft light brown sugar

Pinch of ground cinnamon

Pinch of sea salt

Mint leaves, finely chopped, to serve

POMEGRANATE & LIME

Serves 2

Prep time: 5 minutes plus freezing

Tip the pomegranate seeds onto a baking tray, shake out into an even layer and freeze for 1 hour until solid.

Tip into a food processor, add the lime juice, sugar, cinnamon and salt and blend until fine.

Either serve immediately, with the mint, or tip back into the tray and freeze until you're ready to serve.

Juice of 3 red grapefruit (300ml)

Juice of 1 large orange (150ml)

2 tsp maple syrup or honey

Pinch of ground cardamom

Pinch of sea salt

20g slivered pistachios

GRAPEFRUIT & ORANGE

Serves 2

Prep time: 10 minutes plus freezing

Pour the juices into a baking tray or plastic container (using metal really speeds up the process), stir in the honey, cardamom and salt and freeze for 30 minutes until ice crystals begin to form around the edges.

Use a fork to scrape the crystals into the middle of the liquid, then return to the freezer.

Continue this process every half hour until no liquid remains and you have a dry/fluffy granita. Serve with the pistachios.

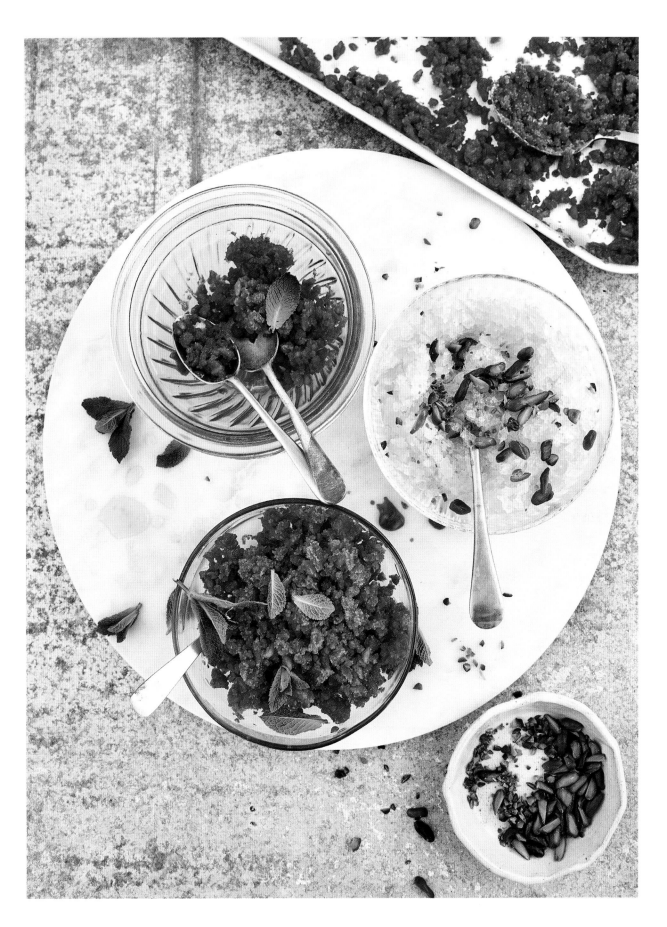

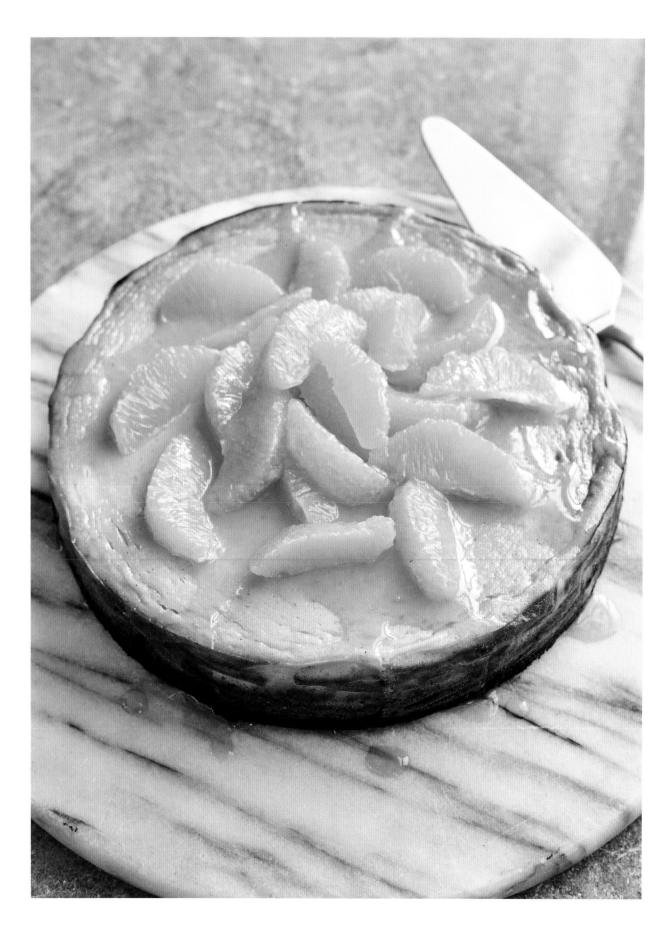

VANILLA CHEESECAKE WITH ORANGE OIL

Serves 8

Prep time: 20 minutes, plus soaking and chilling
Cook time: 45 minutes

I'll be honest, I'm not much of a baker, but I always have this recipe up my sleeve. I adore making this simple dessert because I love cheesecake. Using my secret ingredient makes it far more nutritious and less heavy than dairy, without compromising flavour. The sweet crumb is packed with gorgeous zesty orange and jammy dates. Don't tell your friends that the topping is made of silken tofu before they taste it, then watch their reaction…

Coconut oil, for greasing

For the base
150g cashews
100g pistachios
50g shelled hemp seeds
100g pitted Medjool dates
Finely grated zest of 1 orange

For the filling
150g cashews
500g silken tofu
4 tbsp maple syrup
1 tbsp cornflour
Grated zest and juice of 1 lemon
1 vanilla pod, split lengthways

To serve
2 oranges, segmented
2 tbsp maple syrup
2 tbsp extra virgin olive oil

Preheat the oven to 160°C fan. Grease a 20cm springform cake tin and line with baking parchment.

For the base, put the nuts and hemp seeds into a food processor and blend to a fine powder. Add the dates, orange zest and a pinch of salt and blend again to a coarse crumb. Tip the mixture into the lined tin and use the back of a spoon to press it into the base and sides. Transfer to the oven for 15 minutes.

For the filling, soak the cashews in boiling water for 20 minutes. Drain the cashews and put into a blender with the tofu, maple syrup, cornflour, lemon zest and juice, vanilla seeds and a pinch of salt. Blend on a high speed for 2 to 3 minutes until completely smooth, then pour onto the cooked base.

Bake for 30 minutes until set with a slight wobble in the centre. Turn the oven off, leave the door open slightly and leave to cool completely. Transfer to the fridge and chill for at least 2 hours.

Meanwhile, combine the orange segments, maple syrup and olive oil in a bowl and set aside to infuse.

Serve the cheesecake topped with the orange pieces and drizzled with the olive oil mixture.

Substitutions
Oranges: clementines or other seasonal fruit

MAKING THE MOST OF INGREDIENTS

A common query goes like this: 'I bought sumac for a recipe. It tastes great, but I've no idea how to use it up.' Never leave anything languishing in the cupboard. For more unusual ingredients, here are ideas for what else to do with them.

Artichokes in brine
Chop and add to veggie stir fries with fresh peas and tomatoes.

Baharat/Ras el hanout/Lebanese spice mix
Use to garnish yoghurt, chickpeas and even roasted tomatoes, with garlic and olive oil.

Capers
Use to finish pastas. You can also blend with olive oil, olives and garlic for a quick tapenade.

Caraway seeds
Use toasted on potatoes or carrots. Sauté with fennel, chilli and cumin to start a veggie dish.

Cardamom
Make chai with a teabag, cloves, cinnamon and black pepper.

Chestnuts
Crumble into sautés with garlic and greens.

Chipotle paste
For a cauli bite, use to smother chopped florets, drizzle in oil and roast for 30 minutes.

Cinnamon sticks
Add to broths or hot water with a rooibos teabag as a decaffeinated cinnamon tonic.

Cloves
Add to hot water, lemon and honey for a tea.

Curry leaves
Use to start off any curry or rice, or fry on their own and use to top a curry. Freeze to store.

Gochujang
Add to sauces and stews, like goulash or even ragù, to spice things up with a sweet heat.

Jalapeños
Scatter over a frittata, in scrambled eggs or as a garnish for black beans and tacos.

Miso paste
Add to hot water with greens, beansprouts and mushrooms to make miso soup. Or loosen with water and oil for a stir-fry seasoning sauce.

Mustard seeds
Add to stir fries with ginger and garlic or add to curries with other spices, for tempering and to add an earthy flavour.

Pomegranate molasses
Drizzle over coconut yoghurt or ice cream, add a tablespoon to water instead of cordial for a zesty drink, and use instead of maple syrup as a sweetener in Middle Eastern stews.

Roasted red peppers
Blend with olive oil to create a dip, or throw into the base of passata when making pasta, for a sweet kick.

Sri Lankan curry powder
Use in curries instead of garam masala.

Sumac
Use to finish eggs or jazz up a dip, like hummus or baba ganoush. Add to soup for a zesty tang.

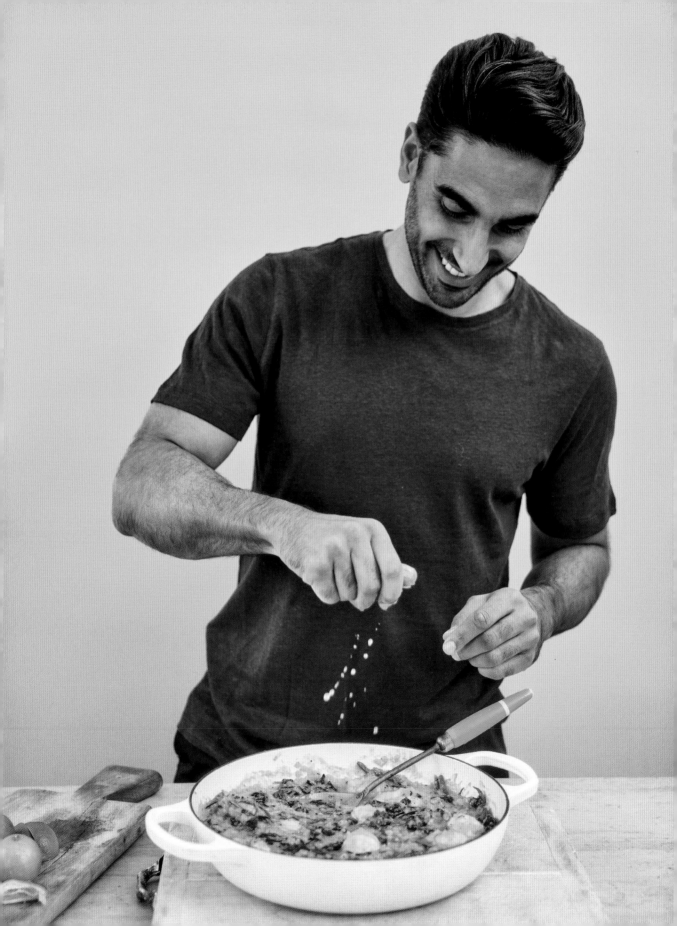

INDEX

COOK'S INDEX

REFERENCES

Govindarajan R, Vijayakumar M, Pushpangadan P. 'Antioxidant approach to disease management and the role of "Rasayana" herbs of Ayurveda'. *Journal of Ethnopharmacology.* 2005 Jun 3; 99(2):165-78. doi: 10.1016/j.jep.2005.02.035. Epub 2005 Apr 26. PMID: 15894123.

Auddy B, Ferreira M, Blasina F, Lafon L, Arredondo F, Dajas F, Tripathi PC, Seal T, Mukherjee B. 'Screening of antioxidant activity of three Indian medicinal plants, traditionally used for the management of neurodegenerative diseases'. *Journal of Ethnopharmacology.* 2003 Feb;84(2-3):131-8. doi: 10.1016/s0378-8741(02)00322-7. PMID: 12648805.

Sproesser G, Ruby MB, Arbit N et al. 'Understanding traditional and modern eating: the TEP10 framework'. *BMC Public Health.* 2019;19(1):1606. Published 2019 Dec 2. doi:10.1186/s12889-019-7844-4.

Gabriel AS, Ninomiya K, Uneyama H. 'The role of the Japanese traditional diet in healthy and sustainable dietary patterns around the world'. *Nutrients.* 2018;10(2):173. Published 2018 Feb 3. doi:10.3390/nu10020173.

Lee J, Pase M, Pipingas A, Raubenheimer J, Thurgood M, Villalon L, Macpherson H, Gibbs A, Scholey A. 'Switching to a 10-day Mediterranean-style diet improves mood and cardiovascular function in a controlled crossover study'. *Nutrition.* 2015 May; 31(5):647-52. doi: 10.1016/j.nut.2014.10.008. Epub 2014 Nov 4. PMID: 25837207.

Wallace TC, Bailey RL, Blumberg JB, Burton-Freeman B, Chen CO, Crowe-White KM, Drewnowski A, Hooshmand S, Johnson E, Lewis R, Murray R, Shapses SA, Wang DD. 'Fruits, vegetables, and health: a comprehensive narrative, umbrella review of the science and recommendations for enhanced public policy to improve intake'. *Critical Reviews in Food Science and Nutrition.* 2020;60(13):2174-2211. doi: 10.1080/10408398.2019.1632258. Epub 2019 Jul 3. PMID: 31267783.

Steer E. 'A cross comparison between Ayurvedic etiology of Major Depressive Disorder and bidirectional effect of gut dysregulation'. *Journal of Ayurveda and Integrative Medicine.* 2019;10(1):59-66. doi:10.1016/j.jaim.2017.08.002.

Guarino MPL, Altomare A, Emerenziani S, Di Rosa C, Ribolsi M, Balestrieri P, Iovino P, Rocchi G, Cicala M. 'Mechanisms of action of prebiotics and their effects on gastro-intestinal disorders in adults'. *Nutrients.* 2020 Apr 9;12(4):1037. doi: 10.3390/nu12041037. PMID: 32283802; PMCID: PMC7231265.

van Loo J, Coussement P, de Leenheer L, Hoebregs H, Smits G. 'On the presence of inulin and oligofructose as natural ingredients in the western diet'. *Critical Reviews in Food Science and Nutrition.* 1995 Nov;35(6):525-52. doi: 10.1080/10408399509527714. PMID: 8777017.

Zhou K. 'Strategies to promote abundance of Akkermansia muciniphila, an emerging probiotics in the gut, evidence from dietary intervention studies'. *Journal of Functional Foods.* 2017; 33:194-201. doi:10.1016/j.jff.2017.03.045.

Peron, Gregorio et al. 'Crosstalk among intestinal barrier, gut microbiota and serum metabolome after a polyphenol-rich diet in older subjects with "leaky gut": The MaPLE trial'. *Clinical Nutrition* (Edinburgh, Scotland) vol. 40,10 (2021): 5288-5297. doi:10.1016/j.clnu.2021.08.027.

Pérez-Jiménez J, Neveu V, Vos F et al. 'Identification of the 100 richest dietary sources of polyphenols: an application of the Phenol-Explorer database'. *European Journal of Clinical Nutrition* 64, S112–S120 (2010). https://doi.org/10.1038/ejcn.2010.221.

Wallace, TC et al. 'Fruits, vegetables, and health: A comprehensive narrative, umbrella review of the science and recommendations for enhanced public policy to improve intake'. *Critical Reviews in Food Science and Nutrition,* vol. 60,13 (2020): 2174-2211. doi: 10.1080/10408398.2019.1632258.

Han Y; Xiao H (2020). 'Whole food-based approaches to modulating gut microbiota and associated diseases'. *Annual Review of Food Science and Technology,* 11(1), annurev-food-111519-014337. doi:10.1146/annurev-food-111519-014337.

McDonald D et al. 'American gut: an open platform for citizen science microbiome research'. *mSystems* vol. 3,3 e00031-18. 15 May. 2018, doi:10.1128/mSystems.00031-18.

Heiman ML, Greenway FL. 'A healthy gastrointestinal microbiome is dependent on dietary diversity'. *Molecular Metabolism,* vol. 5,5 317-320. 5 Mar. 2016. doi:10.1016/j.molmet.2016.02.005.

Huckleberry Y. 'Nutritional support and the surgical patient'. *American Journal of Health-System Pharmacy: AJHP: Official Journal of the American Society of Health-System Pharmacists,* vol. 61,7 (2004): 671-82; quiz 683-4.

Martin-McGill KJ, Bresnahan R, Levy RG, Cooper PN. 'Ketogenic diets for drug-resistant epilepsy'. *Cochrane Database of Systematic Reviews 2020,* Issue 6. Art. No.: CD001903. doi: 10.1002/14651858.CD001903.pub5.

Kelly T et al. 'Low-carbohydrate diets in the management of obesity and type 2 diabetes: a review from clinicians using the approach in practice'. *International Journal of Environmental Research and Public Health,* vol. 17,7 2557. 8 Apr. 2020. doi:10.3390/ijerph17072557.

Kringelbach ML. 'The pleasure of food: underlying brain mechanisms of eating and other pleasures'. *Flavour,* 4, 20 (2015). https://doi.org/10.1186/s13411-014-0029-2.

Plassmann H et al. 'Marketing actions can modulate neural representations of experienced pleasantness'. *Proceedings of the National Academy of Sciences of the United States of America,* vol. 105,3 (2008): 1050-4. doi:10.1073/pnas.0706929105.

Boles DZ et al. 'Can exercising and eating healthy be fun and indulgent instead of boring and depriving? Targeting mindsets about the process of engaging in healthy behaviors'. *Frontiers in Psychology,* vol. 12 745950. 5 Oct. 2021. doi:10.3389/fpsyg.2021.745950.

Turnwald BP, Crum AJ. 'Smart food policy for healthy food labelling: leading with taste, not healthiness, to shift consumption and enjoyment of healthy foods'. *Preventive Medicine,* vol. 119 (2019): 7-13. doi:10.1016/j.ypmed.2018.11.021.

ACKNOWLEDGEMENTS

To my mum, dad, sister and wife whose love and support allow me to chase my ambitions. Thank you for allowing me to pursue what's right in my heart and what I know ultimately makes me happy and healthy.

To my mentors, seniors and closest friends who all have an unwavering confidence in what I do, even when I'm riddled with self-doubt and indecision. Your love and strength of belief is what keeps me moving forward bit by bit.

To my new, incredible publishing team at Ebury, headed up by Lizzy Gray, the photographer David Loftus and the recipe styling crew, the designer Luke Bird, my amazing literary agent, Carly Cook, and Rich Harris, for assisting with recipe creation. Thank you all for elevating my creative work and I sincerely hope that we can continue to champion recipes for delicious and health-supporting food for many years to come.

To Karen Scott. Your work, support and weekly chats have been critical to the success of the business and I'm so lucky you reached out to me all those years ago when I was a one-man band trying to juggle everything. I can't express how grateful I am for you.

To the Doctor's Kitchen team. We are small but powerful and we will have a huge impact.

To my online community of Doctor's Kitchen app users, newsletter subscribers, social media followers. None of this is possible without you and I feel your support and energy.

To the scientists in the field of nutrition, medicine and lifestyle whose work forms the very backbone of everything at Doctor's Kitchen. You are the reason why I can speak confidently about lifestyle medicine and what drives our mission. My love and appreciation to you all.

To all health professionals transforming the way they practice and becoming beacons of a movement that embraces food and lifestyle as medicine. Together we will revolutionise wellbeing and healthcare for the better.

To my patients who teach me as much as I am able to help them. For the most privileged of positions as a doctor and to care for those in their most vulnerable state, I am so grateful.

We all need to take the time to be grateful for our achievements. Whatever you call it – self-love, self-care, self-congratulation – taking a moment to acknowledge ourselves when we've worked hard or achieved a goal supports good mental health. So I also want to thank myself. I know it's slightly strange and not the cultural norm, but I'm the type of person who rarely takes a moment to reflect on my own hard work and dedication.

Rupy. You help millions of people around the world to improve their health one step at a time. You create recipes, write books, release podcasts, mentor, lecture, research and practice medicine. And now you're venturing into the health tech space with your app and the aspiration to help a billion people leverage the medicinal power of food to prevent illness and improve wellbeing. You're doing OK, mate. Pat yourself on the back, keep it up and be grateful.

1

Ebury Press, an imprint of Ebury Publishing
20 Vauxhall Bridge Road, London SW1V 2SA

Ebury Press is part of the Penguin Random House
group of companies whose addresses can be found
at global.penguinrandomhouse.com

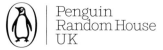

Text copyright © Rupy Aujla 2023
Photography copyright © David Loftus 2023

Rupy Aujla has asserted his right to be identified as the author of
this Work in accordance with the Copyright, Designs and Patents
Act 1988

First published by Ebury Press in 2023

www.penguin.co.uk

A CIP catalogue record for this book is available
from the British Library

ISBN 9781529148831

The authorised representative in the EEA is Penguin Random House
Ireland, Morrison Chambers, 32 Nassau Street, Dublin D02 YH68.

Project Editor: Lisa Pendreigh
Designer: Luke Bird
Photographer: David Loftus
Food and Props Stylist: Libby Silbermann

Colour origination by Altaimage, London
Printed and bound by L.E.G.O. S.p.A., Vicenza, Italy

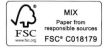

Penguin Random House is committed to a sustainable
future for our business, our readers and our planet.
This book is made from Forest Stewardship Council®
certified paper.

> **"Excellent. I loved that it included a generous amount of vegetables, but they were subtle."**

Madeleine Smith
Madeleine Whiteley
Madlaina Michelotti
Dr Maggie Deytrikh
Maggie Ridehalgh
Maggie Simmons
Maggie White
Maggie Wood
Mairead Bergin
Mandeep Kaur
  Takher-Smith
Marcia Mertens
Maree Burke

Marzena Esposito
Maureen Dunn
Max & Elise Ruijsbroek
May Macdonald
Megan Tarry
Megan Weeding
Melanie Redman
Melanie Seymour
Melanie West
Michele Brough
Michelle Morgan
Mina Mann
Moira Boakes

Kate Hosking
Kate Wisdom
Katharine Bright
Katharine Louise
  D'Arcy
Kathleen Sides
Kathryn Pearce
Kathy Collins
Katie Hill
Katie Taylor
Katy Montague
Kavindra Palaraja
Kay Johnstone
Kay Maloney
Kay Snowdon
Kerry Kerslake
Kim Taylor
Kristin Anderson
Kuljit Paddan

Laetitia Pele
Laura Grant
Laura Rose
Lauren Martin
Lauren Munton
Lauren Wheeler
Leah Hattrell
Leisha Champion
Lesley Crosby
Lesley June
  Stainbank
Lesley Neagle
Liana Fruchtman
  Colas
Lib Khoo
Liesl Popplewell
Lili Dingwall
Lin Sanderson
Linda Davidson
Linda Ferrari
Linda Gray
Linda Guiver
Lindsey Thompson
Lisa Adcock
Lisa Buckley
Lisa Currie
Lisa Mayhew
Liuba Hodgson
Liz Llewellyn

Liz Pearson
Lizzie Robinson
Lorenza Gay
Lori Lauscher
Lorinda Homberger
Lorna Bellamy
Lorna Blythe
Lorraine Munt
Lorraine Spence
Lorraine Surgin
Louise Brewer
Louise Hallam
Louise Jones
Louise Moore

Louise Searson
Louise Simmonds
Louise & Andrew Turl
Lucy, Jack & Babs
  Bennett
Lucy Morrish
Lucy Murray
Lucy Pratt
Lucy Stern
Lyn & Malcolm Walker
Lyndsey Goddard
Lynn Harris
Lynn Murray
Lynne Widdison

> **"A big hit. We would be happy to eat this every day!"**

> **"Incredibly easy, fuss-free and super-tasty."**

Margaret O'Brien
Margaret Reckitt
Mari Craig
Maria Catherine Hulme
Marian Freeman
Marion Collins
Marion Nulty
Marjo de Haas
Mark Garside
Mark Lean
Martine Holmes
Mary Hunter
Mary Stewart
Mary-Elizabeth McNeill

Moira Hardie
Monika Jakimowicz

Nadia Sinovich
Nancy Tzeng
Nancy Van Den Broeck
Naomi Kihams
Natalie Atkins
Natalie Blackburn
Natalie Cook
Natasha Agombar
Neelum Wyman
Neeta Parekh
Nick Jones
Nicki Bennison
Nicki Keyworth
Nicky Rodgers
Nicola Adams
Nicola Askham
Nicola Campbell
Nicola Evered
Nicola Long
Nicola Salzer
Nicola Sochacka
Nicole de Souza
Nilly Jassal
Norman Jubb

> **"It sounded like an odd combination, but it was surprisingly delicious."**

Pablo Rosenthal-Almire
Pam Lockwood